MEDICINE IN SEARCH

OF

MEANING

BY

BILL BAZAN

Caritas Communications
A Division of Word Working, Inc.
5526 West Elmhurst Drive
Mequon, Wisconsin 53092-2010

Bazan, Bill
MEDICINE IN SEARCH OF MEANING
ISBN 0-9668228-2-X

DEDICATION

This book is dedicated to the memory of Dr. Harold Borkowf (1936 – 1995) whose skills and caring brought my children Sammy and Jessie safely into this world.

ACKNOWLEDGMENTS

There are several people that I want to acknowledge for their pivotal role in helping me along the way as I prepared my book. I want to thank the Catholic Health Association of Wisconsin, its president, Sister Rosemary Sabino, and Board of Directors, for allowing me the freedom to pursue the development of the Medicine in Search of Meaning program. I owe a huge debt of gratitude to Sister Rhea Emmer, a friend, colleague, and partner in the development and facilitation of the program. I am profoundly grateful to the many physicians whose time and insight provided my 'looking glass' into the physician world, especially Dr. Glenn Ragalie, Dr. David Weissman, Dr. Steve Sievers, Dr. Maureen Murphy–Greenwood, and the late Dr. Harold Borkowf; and to the many friends and colleagues who have been supportive over the years, including Sister Renee Rose, Dr. Marv Kolb, Dr. Len Scarpinato, Theresa Reagan, Gene Korienek, John Waldbauer, Karen Vernal, John Vishnevsky, Jim Balistreri, and Wally Belau. I want to make a special mention of my friend Dan Dwyer and his wife, Estela Monjo. Dan helped me edit this book and assisted me in processing the experiences of my life for countless hours over bottomless cups of coffee. Finally, I owe deep and everlasting gratitude to Peg Flahive, the mother of our children, and to Sammy and Jessie who continually teach me to be a more loving father.

TESTIMONY FROM PHYSICIANS

"*Medicine in Search of Meaning* is a wonderful, self–reflective book that will help physicians rekindle their passion for medicine and the patients they serve during these times of tumultuous change in the delivery of health care. Bill has brought the business of the heart and soul back into the business of medicine!"

Marvin Kolb, M.D., Medical Director, Kern County Hospital, Bakersfield, CA, and a member of the Quality Leadership Team for the American Hospital Association.

"In his easy, direct style, Bill Bazan offers physicians a way to reawaken the dream that brought all of us into the practice of medicine. He helps physicians bring a deeper sense of meaning and purpose into their world by developing their personal spirituality, thereby, accessing their inner dynamic forces of energy and power. The recipients of this energy are both the patients and the physicians."

Len Scarpinato, D.O., Director of the Family Practice Residency program, All Saints Health System, Racine, Wisconsin.

"Having participated in the first Medicine in Search of Meaning program back in 1992, I realized that Bill Bazan had something substantial to offer to medical practitioners. As one who encouraged him to write, I believe this book will help busy physicians hold their lives still for a time, and will provide an impetus to change, beginning with paying closer attention to the promptings of their inner spirit."

Glenn Ragalie, M.D., pulmonologist at St. Mary's Hospital, Milwaukee, Wisconsin.

"*Medicine in Search of Meaning* offers wonderful insight into the relationship between religion and spirituality. One's faith tradition, and its teachings, prayer forms, and celebrations, are meant to serve one's spiritual nature. This book offers excellent suggestions to health professionals seeking to enrich their clinical experiences and nurture their souls."

David Weissman, M.D., Director of the Palliative Care Program, Medical College of Wisconsin.

PREFACE

Health care is undergoing critical, dynamic transformation. In the midst of the white water rapids of change, stands the physician community. Issues such as autonomy of practice, utilization review, managed care income, malpractice suits, defensive medicine, the business side of practicing medicine, and a seemingly endless stream of meetings, can leave clinical practitioners out in the cold without focus or a sense of meaning. This book challenges physicians to find their bearings during these turbulent times by looking at an inner source of power that is often not acknowledged, much less accessed. In short, we are all on a spiritual journey. If there are differences in this regard, they lie in the fact that some of us are more adept at raising our spiritual journey to a conscious level.

Medicine in Search of Meaning encourages us to be more self–reflective, to hold our lives still, for brief moments, so we can access meaning and purpose deep within our souls. I wrote it because physicians told me that the dreams that led them into medicine have gone to very quiet places inside. Instead of those dreams consciously evolving over time and guiding physicians through their personal and professional lives, they have been largely replaced by feverish activity, fear, worry, anger and depression. As one physician put it so succinctly: "It is as if my heart has been cut out!" To put heart back into the practice of medicine is to learn how to access the power and energy in the very core of our being and release it into a world that often does not welcome such gifts.

After traveling around this country, speaking with and learning from hundreds of physicians, I have been encouraged by them to write. If there is any success to this book, it is due primarily to the many physicians, both in the clinical practice and administrative sides of medicine, who have freely shared their life experiences with me. If *Medicine in Search of Meaning* falls short, the responsibility rests upon my shoulders.

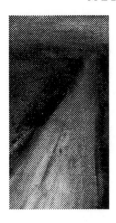

Chapter One

A DEEPER SENSE OF MEANING

"If I don't know where I'm going, any direction will do!"

The physical world can be a magnificent learning environment. It can be a school yard within which, through varied and sundry experiences, we come to know and understand what causes us to grow and what causes us to remain static, what causes us to expand in perspective and increase in depth. In the physical world, we come to discern what nurtures our soul and spirit and what literally depletes our energy. In reality, we soon discover what works and what doesn't work for us. My experience of the traditions of medicine, and in particular of the traditions of the medical practitioner, tells me that the physical, corporeal world of people is where physicians roam, have power, and feel most comfortable.

But what about a world of medicine that is changing so fast that the air is getting sucked out of the balloons of meaning that once gave solace and comfort in the past to countless numbers of physicians? What about a medical culture that is being challenged to rethink and redefine its very purpose for existence? What about the autonomy issues that are being raised by physicians who feel the presence of face-less people – lawyers, insurance utilization review personnel, and health care executives – telling them how to practice medicine in their own examining rooms? What about the pressures coming from outside groups who want physicians to align with them in networks and not with their competitors down the street? What about the fears that accompany physicians who are questioning whether or not they are still relevant for this new age of medicine and its delivery? Finally, what about the physicians who believe medical school and medical training have left them hanging out to dry with little or no formation in the business side of medicine, much less in the human, spiritual side of medical practice; a medical training system that teaches diagnostic skills, vast sums of knowledge and technological development, but precious little on how to handle anger, frustration, bitterness and the demands of change?

Does any of the following sound familiar?

"I have no time anymore – for my family, for my friends, and to take a walk in the park. Things happen so fast ... so many demands on my time ... so little time." (a Family Practitioner)

"I'm getting nervous about my future in medicine. As a specialist in cardiovascular surgery, will I be shut out in a capitated market place? How will financial incentives be structured to account for me in the new health care delivery schemes?" (a Cardiovascular Surgeon)

"Government red tape, regulations, and less part B Medicare payments for my services are just some of the shit–loads of crap that have spoiled it for me! Thank God I've only got a few more years before retirement. The politicians can go to hell in a hand basket as far as I'm concerned." (an Internist)

"Medical malpractice threats and those God–awful premiums every quarter ... give me a break. All I every wanted to do was help women and families deliver kids and be healthy. That's why I went into medicine in the first place." (an Obstetrician/Gynecologist)

"I've noticed today more than yesterday how much division there is among my own colleagues. Everybody seems to be out to protect their own piece of the money tree and the turf that gets the money. That's not why I got into medicine." (a Cardiologist)

During the past ten years, I have spent considerable time working with and conversing with physicians from all parts of the country, but especially in Wisconsin where I live and work. In October of 1992, along with my friend and partner Sister Rhea Emmer, a program called "Medicine in Search of Meaning" was inaugurated. This is a program and a process meant to assist physicians in rediscovering or reconnecting to a deeper sense of meaning and purpose in their clinical practices of medicine. It is a process–oriented program designed for between six and fifteen physicians at a time. Beginning on a Friday evening and going through lunch on Saturday, time is spent by the participants dialoguing around three case studies designed to help them look at and reflect on three specific areas important to their lives: family, patients and peers.

The structure and focus of the program are rather simple. Time is provided for medical colleagues to talk about the dreams that led them into medicine in the first place (as well as what positively and negatively impacts on that dream today). An environment is created wherein physicians talk about the issues and challenges that confront them as persons underneath their roles as physicians. This human or spiritual side of medicine, as countless numbers of physicians have told me, never gets talked about or even considered. "Medicine in Search of Meaning" becomes an opportunity for participants to share their own thoughts and to listen to what their peers have to say about this personal, spiritual side of medicine. As facilitators, Rhea and I assist in focusing the dialogue process with an occasional teaching from one of us on the applications of spirituality to what is being said at the time.

The content of this book arose out of my own listening to and sharing with physicians. Several physicians strongly encouraged me to write about the ideas and experiences talked about both in the program itself as well as in private, in–depth conversations in which they engaged with me. All the case studies and interviews I will be sharing with you in the course of this book are real, only the names used are fictitious.

Opening to the Spiritual Dimension

Each and every one of us, no matter what we do in life, are involved in a spiritual journey that weaves its path through the mine–fields and hard knocks of experience as well us through the joys and loves of everyday life. I describe this spiritual journey as a process of coming to power and discovering meaning – a power and meaning beyond anything my mind could manufacture all by itself. Spirituality in this context can be described as a powerful inner force we are born with, developmental in nature, that moves us toward wholeness. It is different from religion. Religion is defined by the beliefs, tenets, and liturgical expressions specific to a particular tradition. Most religions arose out of a community's desire to bond and bind together around a particular set of beliefs connected to and derived from the teachings of a great prophet or teacher. Judaism, Roman Catholicism, Protestantism, Islamism, and all the other "isms" that characterize religious belief and tradition are meant, I believe, to serve the spirituality of its members. Simply put: our religion is meant to serve our spirituality, not vice–versa. What we all share in common is a spiritual nature, not always a religious tradition. This book will focus on applying spirituality to the practice of medicine – its purpose is to accompany readers on their spiritual journeys, sometimes evoking, sometimes provoking, but always with the intention of Bill Bazan being a fellow traveler on this journey. I would like to share a part of one particular interview I had with a physician:

Jake: I quit going to church when I entered medical school. I really just grew tired of going to Mass every Sunday and listening to a boring sermon by a priest who always seemed to be asking for money. Religion just wasn't relevant to me. All the way through my medical training and all the way up to the establishment of my practice, I had little or nothing to do with Catholicism. My wife and I were married in the church and my two kids were baptized there. Except for Christmas, Easter and maybe one or two other special occasions, I didn't participate at all – my wife and kids did, but not me. As I got a little older, and I thought wiser, I would engage in great philosophical debates about papal infallibility, the Catholic Church's teachings on birth control and contraceptive procedures, and why women could not be ordained. My medical peers would generally agree with my position. For some unknown reason, I began to get angry at the Church – that seemed to carry over to the sisters who own the Catholic hospital that I practice in. I just couldn't buy into that ethical crap that seemed to define Catholic hospitals.

Bill: What changed you? You don't seem so angry today.

Jake: Along the way, about two years ago, my oldest daughter developed leukemia. Aggressive treatment was needed to save her life. As I sat alone at her bedside while she slept, I kept asking God to help save this little girl. I bargained with Him saying, "I'll go back to church if only you'll save my little girl." This form of blackmail didn't work. My daughter got worse, not better. One night after responding to an emergency room call, I decided to stop in to see how she was doing. As I sat there holding her little hand, she looked over at me and said, "Daddy, don't worry. You'll feel better soon. Take care of yourself. I'll be fine because I know you and mommy love me!" When she said that I started to cry and could not stop for the longest time. I thought to myself about how rich and meaningful my little girl's life was in contrast to my own. For all my knowledge, diagnostic skills and the like, I felt like a shell of a man – real empty inside. As my daughter's illness went into remission and she got better, I started to go back to church every Sunday but I still felt empty inside. Then one day I got it. What I needed was not something outside of me, doing this or that, reading this or that. What I needed to pay attention to was something I have now come to call my spiritual center – the part of me where meaning and purpose come from.

Bill: Where does your religion come in, if anywhere, these days?

Jake: Once I began to listen to what's inside of me and not blame everyone from the Pope to my parish priest, my Catholic faith began to give me a way of expressing what's inside and a way of thanking God.

To argue whether religion is more important than spirituality or spirituality than religion is like trying to solve the question whether the chicken or the egg came first. It's really academic. For many people, myself and Jake included, it is often the spiritual issues in our lives we do not confront and respond to effectively that cause us to feel empty inside. Money, status, religion do not compensate for failing to listen to the spiritual dimensions of our lives.

One of the major components involved in responding to the spiritual dimensions of our life is an understanding of the role our own soul and ego (strategic mind or personality) play along the pathways of our life. A thread that is woven through this book is a belief that meaning and purpose evolve in our life when our ego is aligned with our soul in harmonious concert. Our soul becomes the receptacle of personal power in our life – the place deep within us that is our source of power and energy. This inner source of power is available and accessible whenever we consciously choose to tap into it. It is this inner energy that enables us to process what is happening in our life and to make sense out of it. It is that inner sanctuary where we take our anger, hurt, blame and bitterness in order to learn from them. It is here, in the recesses of our soul, that we find a safe haven to reflect and talk to ourselves, where we sort out and learn from the lessons that our life is holding out for us. It is here, at our spiritual center, where conflicts are transformed into opportunities for new growth, where seeming despair and emptiness are changed into learning experiences of hope, and where we connect with our Higher Power, our God, the Love of the Universe or whatever we choose to call that Entity.

As we come into an awareness that we possess this personal power in our spiritual center, then it is a short distance to realize everyone else has the same gift – a gift that is quite literally a birthright, a condition of being a human being. Along the path of our life with others, we will connect with the sense that this gift has set up a special relationship of energy between ourselves and other people. This special relationship and its being lived out respectfully and consciously is what I call the lived experience of relational power, that is, the capacity to nurture and sustain personal/professional relationships. The ability to do this is built upon the premise that we have power with others (relational power), not over others (unilateral power). As a physician, it could mean being responsible with patients, not just for them; seeing patients as teachers of medical practice (a receiving), not just as a challenging case with which to apply technological and diagnostic skills (a giving only). The relational expression of power and the unilateral expression of power can cause tension points to arise in the life of a physician who has been trained in one of the most unilaterally powerful institutions in the world – medical school and training.

This book is an attempt to augment what medical schools and medical training simply do not do: raise awareness for the clinical practitioner of the spiritual, human side of medicine and assist the practitioner in developing the skills necessary to live into the spiritual dimensions of life, both personally and professionally. I hope it will challenge you enough for you to say: "I think I know where I want to go with my life and any direction simply will not do!" To quote a physician friend, "If I had spent only a fraction of the time and energy that I put into developing my career from the start of medical school to the present on processing the spiritual issues of my life, I wonder what could have been." The question is not one of surrendering to the past and the what ifs of personal history, but one of the present moment and a willingness to start from wherever we are. When that happens, we can plan a direction. The beauty of the spiritual journey is that it starts wherever and whenever we choose to allow it to happen.

Case Study and Reflections

"When does your spiritual quest as a physician begin?
With standard answers or fresh questions?"

Be totally honest for a moment: In the context of the current circumstances of your life, are you happy being where you are today? What aspects of your life are you not happy or content with? Name them. (Pause) Whatever you have just named, either off the top of your head or in quiet reflection, are they places in your personal experience where you need to ask fresh questions and respond with a new mind set. These are the places, the rich fabrics of your life, that need the attention of your soul. These are the starting points for beginning or deepening your spiritual journey. Wishing you were not exactly where you are today is to miss a golden opportunity for renewed meaning.

A case study

Cathy is a 37–year–old internist, married for 10 years, with three children. Her husband works for a plumbing contractor. Cathy loves her work. Her relationship with her husband has grown stagnant over the past three or four years. Cathy cites lack of intellectual stimulation and emotional immaturity as reasons for her lack of interest in staying married. Her children are the main reasons for staying married. After a typically long day that starts with hospital rounds at 7:30 a.m. and her final clinic appointment at 5:30 p.m., Cathy comes home to her television–watching husband and three children whom the nanny is more than willing to surrender to mom! Supper, a little time with the children before bed time, and some reading of professional journals leaves little time for anything else. Cathy and her husband sleep in separate rooms. She is asleep by 10:30. Her husband stays up to watch Jay Leno. Recently, Cathy has been finding excuses to spend time with an equally unhappily married physician at the clinic. She has been calling home two, sometimes three, evenings a week to say she has meetings and medical emergencies to attend. She and her male physician friend have begun a romantic relationship.

Self–Reflection

What area of your life is not working too well right now? Marriage? Relationships? Children? Work? Colleagues? Changes in the health care delivery system? Insurance companies? Law suits? Referral sources? Internal politics at the clinic or hospital? Utilization review specialists? Fear of dying? Loss of a patient? Financial reversals?

Stagnant income? Jealousy or envy? Medical skill or knowledge erosion? Fear of whatever? Addictive behavior of any sort? Poor health or disease? Aging? Anything else you can think of?

You are exactly where you need to be. The point to all of this is: Each and every one of us is exactly where we need to be in our life's journey right now. All the concerns, conflicts and problems presented to us are part and parcel of our life's assignment – no matter how much we deny it. Whenever we take the time to hold our life still for a while and ask new and fresh questions around any of these issues, we will be in a learning mode.

We literally have the capacity to turn habitually enslaving experiences into freeing and liberating opportunities for new growth. This can happen anytime we consciously allow the power of our inner spirit (soul) to accept what is and to learn from it, rather than deny and avoid that which is difficult and distasteful. Meaning and purpose evolve from asking fresh questions about what is not working too well in our life right now. The mind can have the tendency to rationalize and deny. The soul accepts what is and runs with it much like my children do with their favorite bedtime animals. Our soul delights in the present moment's opportunity for deepening life and enriching meaning.

What are your experiences trying to teach you? Once we have struggled with acknowledging our demons, the parts of ourselves we do not see but which drain us of energy, vitality and meaningfulness, they begin to lose power. By asking ourselves what our challenging experiences are trying to teach us, we can begin to move from feelings of being trapped and hopeless to feelings of freedom and hope. In our soul, perhaps, lies the power to create a desired future for ourselves. If we believe we are exactly where we need to be in our life, with all the assignments being presented to us, then perhaps we are in a place to make choices that will assist us along our spiritual journey. After spending some quality time with Cathy, she made a remarkable discovery. "It's not my husband, is it? He is just an easy target of blame and rationalizing of my behavior. I may end up getting a divorce at some moment in my life, but it will not be before I begin to look at my own life and to take some deeper responsibility. I guess I always wanted him to change, not me." I close this essay with a quotation I shared with Cathy – from a Tibetan Buddhist teaching I read somewhere:

"Confess all your hidden faults! Approach that which you find repulsive! Whoever you think you cannot help, help them! Anything you are attached to, let go of it! Go to places that scare you, like cemeteries! Sentient beings are limitless as the sky, be aware! Find the Buddha inside yourself!" (Find a loving God inside of you!)

Your thoughts along the way

(Take a moment to write down any thoughts or insights you want to remember.)

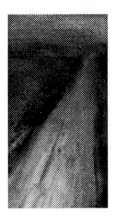

Chapter Two

THE POWER OF SOUL: THE FORGOTTEN DIMENSION

Have you ever found yourself, as I have, hearing or reading a certain word and dismissing its significance because you think you already know what it means? And what if you later discover that the word is one of the most important words you could ever learn about? One such word is soul. Here is a word I have heard since I was a little boy being taught the Baltimore Catechism by Sister Mildred in third grade. Here is a word – in truth a concept, a reality, and so much more – I have heard about and have had little understanding of for many years. Usually in the context of some religious discussion or funeral eulogy or Sunday sermon, the word soul gets bantered about quite fluently and elegantly. "Your immortal soul ... heaven, hell or someplace in between ... may his soul rest in peace ... may her soul and the souls of all the faithfully departed rest in peace. Amen." My early experience of this word soul has been associated with funerals, fire and brimstone sermons, and catechism classes.

It has taken me a long time to associate soul, and whether or not I have one, much less my experience of one, with something concrete, positive and usable in everyday living. Moving beyond (but not necessarily discarding) my childhood beliefs about the nature and function of my soul, I now see more and more clearly that an experience of soul is vital if meaning and purpose are to evolve in my life. As I began to open up my own mind and heart to newer and deeper understandings of what soul means – and my soul in particular – I discovered a whole new way of experiencing my life. Focus, deeper consciousness of real power in my life, and a renewed sense of meaning all came to me as gifts as I began to let go of stereotypical beliefs around the idea and experience of soul.

Has medicine lost its soul?

Following is an excerpt from an interview with a 38–year–old physician who is part of an Emergency Medicine group that contracts out its services to hospitals....

Bill: You were telling me about your experiences in medical school and residency around the issue of balance and where your time and energy was spent. Say more if you would.

Pat: Science was our god in medical school. The way we paid homage to this god was to thoroughly memorize, digest and spew back what we were learning. I felt great doing this because I was successful at it. Sleep and a healthy diet were things of distant memory! My mind and my capacity for deductive reasoning were growing by leaps and bounds. By the time I got into residency, patients were diagnostic challenges that afforded me the chance to apply my scientific knowledge and to learn even more. Nowhere along the line was the word soul uttered, much less ways of taking care of ourselves. It was only when I got into private practice that I started to wonder what I was missing out on. My marriage failed, I began to put on weight ... You know the scenario – I felt like a piece of meat that everyone seemed to want a piece of. I felt just horrible inside – like nothing was there. I was living alone and never did like the person I was living with ... me. I began to question whether or not I should get out of medicine, try something else. What the hell would I have to lose? I really needed to know what happened to my dreams that led me into medicine in the first place. Where did they go anyway? I really felt let down by my training – not in being a doctor, but in becoming a well–rounded person? Where do I start that journey?

Later on in the interview with Pat, he shared something rather profound. "I feel like I've sold out in the process of becoming the doctor others wanted me to be. Never once, until recently, did I ever even think of asking the question: what kind of doctor do I want to be? Once I began to ask that question, my dreams, values and moral concerns began to surface, slowly but surely." What I would add to Pat's comment is this: the place he listens for what nourishes his life is his soul, the source of power that is available to him whenever he chooses to access it. This is the purpose of this chapter: to understand with greater clarity where our real power is, and how to access it and use its energy for growth into meaning and purpose. The context within which this discussion will evolve is that of the physicians who, like Pat, struggle to find deeper meaning and purpose, who desire a more balanced life, and who have come to believe that science and the traditional medical model of practicing medicine is not the be all and end all.

Soul and personality

The decisions we make in this world are the frames of reference that determine whether we continue to grow or remain static, whether we are becoming who we are meant to be or becoming who others want us to be. Who am I? and Who am I becoming? are essential life–long questions. To assist in opening up these two questions for further discussion and reflection, a meaningful understanding of the differences between the life of our soul and the life of our personality would be helpful. (Please note: for purposes of this book, descriptions and lived experiences will be more helpful than definitions in talking about the life of the soul and the life of the personality.

Have you ever found yourself in a situation where you either experienced someone not hearing what you said or you yourself did not really hear what someone else said to you? (I recently heard a wonderful, humorous story that illustrated this point. Two elderly couples were seated together in a retirement home. Without mincing words, Clara asked Maude: "Do you and Joe still have mutual orgasm?" Maude thought for a moment and replied: "No, I think we still have State Farm!") Have you ever tried to describe what steak tastes like to someone who has never eaten it or what an orgasm feels like to someone who has never experienced it? It may be just as difficult to describe the concept and experience of soul. When I use the word soul, I mean the deepest part of me that makes us who we are, that life force or energy that connects us to whatever or whomever we call our Higher

Power. Our soul or inner spirit is the part of us that intrinsically defines us as special, unique, and one–of–a–kind. We are born with a soul, a life force, a power that can quite literally impel us towards wholeness, meaning and profound purpose. Our soul is the primary resource that reveals to us who we are. The key to understanding the soul is to learn ways of accessing and experiencing its power, staying connected to it during our life's journey and allowing it to become the primary mover and shaker in our life.

Our personality, on the other hand, is the part of us we were born into, that we live within. It is that with which we relate to the world around us in a visible way and that within which we will eventually die. To be a human being and to have a personality are one and the same. Our personality, much like our body, is the vehicle of our evolution in this lifetime. (For my purposes here, I will be using ego and strategic mind in somewhat interchangeable ways with personality.) Our decisions and their consequences are the gasoline that fuels our evolution in this lifetime. Whether these decisions will nurture or retard our growth and development on any level – physical, emotional, spiritual, or intellectual – is dependent on the choices we make. Choice is always the key. The question remains: where are our choices grounded and with what are they aligned? I believe that the responses we make to this two–pronged question determine whether or not real meaning and purpose evolve in our life.

In order to draw a clearer distinction between the life of our soul and the life of our personality, I submit the following: our personality generates power by controlling our experiences, while our soul generates power through the experiences that life presents. There is a gigantic difference. To illustrate this point, for a moment, bring to mind a difficult, conflict–filled situation in your life, one that involves another person close to you, a colleague, a spouse, or a good friend. It might even be a clinical situation that is causing you consternation. After the initial encounter, perhaps anger or fear begins to set in. No matter what emotions or thoughts arise, usually one of two things begin to happen: either we focus our attention externally, in terms of blaming, rationalizing, or accusing (the dynamics of ego) or internally, in terms of listening to what this experience is trying to teach us (the dynamics of soul). Our ego tries to "protect" us by controlling the situation with defense mechanisms. Our soul tries to assist our growth and development through teaching us what we need to learn at this moment in time. As always, we choose which path to take.

Letting go of control

"A tale of two cities, each of whom wants to have life."

October 10, 1992, was an important date for Sister Rhea Emmer and I. Rhea, a member of the Congregation of St. Agnes, a religious community of women based in Fond du Lac, Wisconsin, and I were about to embark on our new venture "Medicine in Search of Meaning." At 6:00 p.m. that Friday evening, 14 practicing physicians from St. Mary's Hospital in Milwaukee were going to be coming through the doors of Conference Room A at the Wyndham hotel in downtown Milwaukee. They would be the very first participants to experience our program. Nine months of planning, worrying, wondering and hoping were coming down to a 6:00 pre–program reception. I remember that time as if it were yesterday. I was standing in the hotel lobby around 4:30 wondering to myself: "What in the hell have I gotten myself into now?" I was afraid that what Rhea and I were about to do would bomb badly. (The dynamics of my ego operating...) I flashed back to a time in 8th grade when I felt that same feeling. In front of hundreds of people during the finals of the city of Madison Spelling Bee competition, I was asked to spell the word "insouciance." Of all the words I memorized, this was not one of them! What to do? "Fake it," I remembered telling myself. "I..N..S..O..U..T..I..A...N..C..E" I weakly said. A huge groan came from my grade school cheering section. "I let St. Bernard's down!" I thought as I meekly left the stage. I told myself, "I don't think the judges liked me very much. The others got such easy words." (Again, the dynamics of my ego rationalizing why I was eliminated from the Bee.)

Well, here I was, feeling like the clock was turned back 40 years and I was a little boy again. Fourteen physicians, who were giving up a Friday night and half of Saturday, were going to experience a bomb of a program. (Can you see how my mind was creating a scenario for failure before the fact?) Even at 6'7" in height I felt small. Just about every self–doubt that my mind could muster came to the forefront. I just knew this weekend would be a flop.

"Where in the hell was Rhea? She always seemed to be the steady one – cool under pressure. That's it! I'll wait for her to arrive at the hotel, we'll talk it out, and it will be okay!" Two Diet Pepsis later, I spotted Rhea. She looked at me and with the honesty I have come to respect her for said: "I'm really nervous. I wonder how these doctors will accept me being a former nurse and all?" Taken aback, I blurted out: "That's not what I wanted to hear from you. I wanted you to be so self–assured that we could glide into our opening session at 7:00 without any doubts whatsoever, knowing that our brainchild would be a hit!" (What I was really thinking, but did not say was: "Don't give me that shit, Rhea. Get a hold of yourself. Don't fade out on me now. I don't need to hear about your doubts – mine are enough for the two of us!")

Then something wonderful began to happen. I do not remember which one of us said it, but the following thought was expressed: "If we truly believe in what we are doing, then we must ground ourselves in that belief as we go into Conference Room A." We reminded ourselves that our personalities, our egos, would try to control the situation. If the program failed, it would be the doctors' fault. Our egos would try to take credit if the program succeeded and would blame someone or something else if it failed. Rhea and I both realized then and there that our souls, our own spirits, needed to take the lead, not our personalities. Our souls, and those of the participants, would be empowered the more we let go of trying to make something happen that would conform to our expectations. The more our personalities tried to influence the outcome, the less our souls would be present to the souls of the participants. Real power and energy for everyone involved would come through the experience as it unfolded. Letting go of the fear, the control and the subtle belief that we could manipulate and produce a desired effect if only we would do this or that, or say this or that at the right time, was becoming our soul's learning. (My mind, my ego unaligned with my soul, tries to control the situation because it wants to protect me from feeling bad or fearful.) What was surfacing for us then and there was the very foundation of our program, that is, every person born into this world has a soul, an inner teacher if you will, that will teach whatever lessons we need to learn if only we access it and allow it to do its thing. An unaligned ego that is not soul–driven will lead us further and further away from the very thing we wanted to create – a learning environment where our inner teacher (soul) becomes the primary teacher, the real power and energizer in our life. Soul power in action is learning to access the inner power and energy with which we are born, listening to its promptings, and actively living out what we hear. And yet, during that time in the lobby of the hotel, my ego was willing to sell out and give in to my fears and anxieties. That place in time continues to be a defining moment for me as it reminds me of the vital importance of soul listening and soul action with an aligned ego. My real power is indeed generated through my experiences, not by controlling them.

Soul listening: A true story

I have discovered that it is far easier to learn more about something when I've had an experience of it. For example, once we've tasted pumpkin pie, we are more likely to choose pumpkin pie when ordering dessert. We could read every recipe book from now until the cows come home and we would not know what pumpkin pie tasted like. If, however, we actually put a piece in our mouth, swallowed it, and liked how it tasted, we would be more likely to choose pumpkin pie when the opportunity presented itself. It's really that simple when applied to the nature and experience of our soul. Here is a true story of a physician who received a taste of his soul's presence by actively listening to what his insides were telling him about how to respond in a crisis situation filled with profound human drama. Listening became the instrument for accessing his soul's power. It all happened in the blink of an eye. This is an actual account of a physician from a small midwestern town who shared his soul–story during a "Medicine in Search of Meaning" program:

Nothing like this has ever happened to me before in my 12 years of pediatrics. After a typically hectic day that saw me see 30 patients, I was welcoming the chance to get home and see my family – maybe even watch a movie on TV.

Right after supper, and before I could get the video tape that my wife rented in to the VCR, the hospital paged me to come immediately to the emergency room. One of my patients, a three–month old baby girl, had died at home. The cause of death was determined to be SIDS (Sudden Infant Death Syndrome).

When I arrived, the parents were understandably in shock and, especially the mother, quite hysterical. The father of the baby spotted me first and angrily approached me – almost as if he was going to blame me for what happened to his daughter. "Why did this have to happen to my little girl?" he shouted.

I tried to remain calm, but my insides were churning. A part of me thought about being defensive and telling him it wasn't my fault, but I did not do that. Instead, I urged him to sit down for a moment while I talked to the ER doctor about the circumstances that she was able to ascertain from the paramedics and the couple themselves.

The ER doctor explained that after supper, the father and the little girl were sitting on the living room recliner – the girl resting on his chest with her face buried on his chest. The mother had gone out grocery shopping. Both the father and the little girl fell asleep in the recliner. When the mother returned around 7:30, the father heard the door latch open and he woke up only to discover that his little baby was not breathing. The mother immediately called 911. The paramedics tried to resuscitate the girl, but to no avail. The mother went into shock and the father got angry and started to blame himself for what happened.

After listening to the doctor recall the events of the evening, I went back to the waiting room. Almost immediately the father came up to me again, and in a loud voice with tears streaming down his cheeks said: "Why did this have to happen? It is all my fault. My little baby died on my chest!" He kept repeating that his little girl had died on his chest.

After a few seconds had elapsed, I caught my own breath, looked him straight in the eye and spoke: "I don't know why your daughter died, but she did not die alone. She went to heaven listening to your heartbeat. The last thing she felt was the comfort and love of her father."

You could have heard a pin drop in the hotel's conference room that night as fourteen other physicians listened intently to the pediatrician's recounting of this experience. I was struck – as were the others present that night – that this was a beautiful account of soul–listening and what can happen when we are connected to the power of the soul.

Later on, the pediatrician added that the father became less agitated and angry right after hearing this beautiful response. The father and mother of the dead girl felt great comfort because of the way this pediatrician responded to them – non–clinically, but with genuine human listening.

As the evening progressed, several of the physicians commented on similar experiences in their respective clinical practices. As a group, they acknowledged that medical school did not prepare them for this aspect of the life of the soul at work. One physician put it this way: "Sometimes I can't cure or prevent a catastrophe like a SIDS death, but I am able to be present in a listening and caring way. That is sometimes very hard for me because I am not used to doing that. Most of the time I would call the hospital chaplain down to handle the situation."

There are no cookie cutter answers to the human side of medicine. One size does not fit all. The soul life of a physician comes to center stage in the clinical practice of medicine when there is an acknowledgement that there is in fact a soul to be brought forth. What do we do when we, as physicians, find ourselves in inhumane situations with patients that demand more than clinical, medical expertise and responses can offer?

Case Study and Reflections

"What medical school forgot: the business of the soul"

A physician practicing internal medicine recently wrote me and posed two penetrating, challenging questions that he is wrestling with: "How do I access the power and energy of my soul in times of need? How do I nurture my soul for empowerment and integration into my clinical practice?" These questions followed an in–depth conversation among several physicians and me about how difficult it is to counter the traditional model of medicine within which physicians are educated and formed. Through all the years of medical school, internship, residency and ongoing education, there is little or no focus on how physicians go about "doing the business of the soul."

Case study

Jason P. is a busy family practice physician, serving not only insured patients at a clinic staffed by five physicians, but also an uninsured patient base at a clinic located at a homeless shelter. He is married, with no children, and has been practicing medicine for eight years. In addition, he is a frequent guest lecturer at a local medical school.

Jason's life is almost totally focused on medicine, with a disintegrating marriage to prove it. (Jason told me he was a "good soldier, one that his professors and mentors would be proud of!") What once was his life's passion was turning into an addiction that had made his life both within and outside of medicine unmanageable. Jason shared on several occasions that he couldn't change – this was what he was – a practicing physician trying to make a difference in his world. He was to experience a defining moment that would change the course of his life's path, not only in medicine, but also personally.

A frequent visitor to the homeless shelter, a young man in his mid–twenties, came to the clinic to see Jason. It was closing time, 9:30 on Friday night. Jason was fatigued at the end of a particularly hectic work week. He snapped at the young man, "Charlie, can't you see that we're closing shop. It's not as if you had anything pressing going on. Why in the hell wait until now to come to the clinic? I'll be back Monday night if it's important to see me. Otherwise, someone else will be in tomorrow morning." Charlie left abruptly.

Later that night Charlie was found dead of a self–inflicted gunshot wound. His medical history indicated that he was dying of the AIDS virus. Jason never knew that until Monday night.

Self Reflection

You can give and receive love.
Learn to pay attention to what has heart and meaning. As healers, we can open ourselves up to the "soulfulness of experience" wherein each encounter becomes a moment of allowing our hearts to be deeply touched and moved by life. Over time and unconsciously, Jason's heart had begun to close itself off from feeling the "soulfulness" of the present moment. Patients became nameless, faceless people who needed something from him. Little did he know until Charlie came into his life rather abruptly that he also needed the life of others to keep meaning and purpose alive. Jason's learning: only the open heart of a healer can give and receive love. As a by–product of that energetic interchange and openness, meaning is discovered. The physician's spiritual path is made clearer. The journey is deepened. Healing happens to the healer.

Your soul can create balance. Perhaps the work of our soul is to find and remove whatever gets in the way of us being who we are? Sometimes, and I hear this from physicians themselves, practicing medicine, seeing patients, doing research, making hospital rounds, going to clinical conferences, being on call – can immunize them from the need to connect deeply and consciously with who they are in their souls. Work takes over, with rewards of its own, on a spiritual and mundane level. Without the balancing force of the soul, the very work that gives rewards soon begins to take them away. A line is crossed when balance goes out the window and work for work's sake takes over. One wise person in my life termed this phenomenon as "unrecognized powerlessness." Our life becomes out of control and unmanageable and we don't even know it! Traditional medicine calls this being dedicated. Jason now calls it stupid.

What is it that only you bring? Charlie's death caused Jason to raise several questions for himself that are worth sharing here: What in your current practice of medicine needs to change in order for deeper meaning and purpose to evolve? Where has your spirit gone – a spirit that once valued each encounter of your medical practice as a gift? If medical school has trained you and given you the tools, experience and education to be a successful physician, what is it that only you can bring to your practice of medicine? And a question that I pose: What is your tolerance level for silence in your life, that is, your capacity for being alone to nurture the life of your soul for integration into your daily life?

Your thoughts along the way

*(Take a moment to write down any thoughts
or insights you want to remember.)*

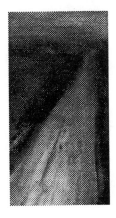

Chapter Three

DISCOVERNG AND NURTURING MEANING

Imagine someone you know and respect stopping you and asking the age-old question, "Who are you?" Stop and reflect a moment – what would you say right off the bat without hesitating at all? What would you say after a thoughtful pause? "Who am I?" is the perennial question of identity that confronts us all initially in our teenage years and later on as our life goes through its various stages of growth and development. There are primary and secondary sources that can reveal our identity to us. Using a spiral as a visual aid, I will be inviting you into another way of looking at the life of the soul and the personality (ego), when they are aligned and not aligned. I suggest that meaning and purpose are discovered and nurtured when the life of our soul (internal focus) and the life of our personality (external focus) are in alignment. One area is not more important than the other. The reason I refer to the life of the soul as the primary source of identity is because it is foundational and integral to giving life (meaning and purpose) to our personality. What we do, then, does not shape our soul. It is indeed the other way around. The life of our personality is manifested in what we do – which changes frequently over time. The life of our soul (who we are intrinsically) does not change as much as it evolves over time into greater clarity and consciousness. The more we learn to access the life of our soul in relationship to what we do, the more meaning and purpose will grow – as well as a renewing sense of hope and vitality emerging in our life.

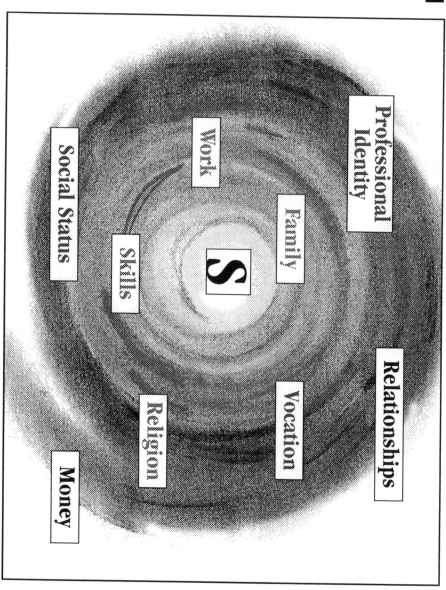

Fig. 3:1

The Spiral Teaching

The life of the soul is represented in the spiral (see fig. 3:1) as a capital S located in the center. This "S" refers to the soul, our true inner self that makes us unique, the core of who we are. This is the deepest part of us, the part that no one can diminish or destroy unless we allow them to do so. Herein lies the center of our spiritual power and energy that impel us towards wholeness, deeper meaning and purpose in life. This "S" forms the bedrock of our personal worth, which connects us to the love of the universe – to our Higher Power which is our God.

As we begin to move outward from the "S" and start to name the secondary sources that describe who we are, we discover such things as job, vocation in life, family, relationships, social status, and financial resources. The list could go on and on with each person having a somewhat different mix of secondary identifications that could be placed on the outer arcs of the spiral. The closer these secondary sources of power and identity are to the center "S" the more integral and important they are in our life. The less important sources are further out from the "S". The key point here is: what energizes and gives meaning to what we do is the "S". The more consciously connected we are to it, the more energy and meaning we experience. The paradox is: the concrete, real situations of our life can provide the context within which to listen and access the power of the "S".

Another facet of the secondary sources of power in our life resides in a rather simple fact: secondary sources can be taken away, diminished, lost, threatened and/or changed. We do not have absolute control of them. Sometimes we have little or no say over these secondary sources. Death, for example, can take a loved one from us. A malpractice suit that is lost in the courts can cause a physician's reputation to be tarnished. Our house could burn down, our spouse could divorce us, the stock market could do irreparable damage to our financial portfolio, etc., etc., etc. If meaning and purpose are only grounded in those areas and suddenly they are gone, then what happens? Where is our life grounded now? If our identity is grounded exclusively in what we do (the secondary sources of power) and some of them are diminished or taken away, then what happens to us? The point here is simply this: the life of the soul needs to be the groundswell and bedrock giving life and meaning to what we do or what we own or with whom we are in relationship.

The Spiral Teaching: A Case Study

Following is a case study illustrative of the spiral teaching...

One indisputable fact has emerged for me as I travel around the country speaking and working with physician groups – the vast majority, if not all, of physicians I've met and talked with have been taught throughout their medical school training that their primary source of power as a physician rests in knowledge acquisition, skill development and diagnostic capacity. Nothing is taught or discussed in regard to their souls or spiritual centers. There is literally no balance created between the rational, scientific thought processes of the mind and the creative, meaning-generating life of the soul. Medical students are left to pick this up on their own. One particular interview I conducted with a family practice physician, who was married and the father of two young children, was consistent with many other physician responses to the issues around the primary and secondary sources of meaning/identity.

Pete: You asked me to provide an overview of my medical school and residency experience. Pressure, competition, memorization and lack of sleep! How about that as a quick overview? Everything, and I mean everything for me, was geared toward knowledge and skill acquisition. While this is obviously vital if I wanted to practice medicine competently, little or nothing was taught us about the person applying the knowledge or using the skill. No one even taught us much about the business side of medical practice, much less about how my soul worked and how meaning is actually accessed. Power as a physician comes from knowledge, skill acquisition, and diagnostic capability. Those are the things I will have to leverage in the real world if I am to make it successfully. That is my identity and the basis of my worth as a person.

Bill: Tell me, Pete, in your own words, what you now understand when applying the spiral concepts to your own experience.

Pete: First of all, I am slowly but surely coming to see that I am more than what I do – more than just a practitioner of medicine. This internal change of mind set continues to be difficult for me to accept. I'm 43 years old and for all those 43 years it has been pounded into me that I am what I do. Medical school and residency reinforced that belief and instilled it more deeply into my thinking. I still feel that I am on a treadmill, churning out patient after patient. That spiral image has caused me to wonder whether or not I have bailed out on my original dream that got me started in medicine way back when.

Bill: You said "original dream." Do you think that was coming from your soul back then?

Pete: I really think so, now that I think about it. You know, I felt real energized – full of piss and vinegar way back then. Nothing was going to stop me from being a physician just like my father. When I announced to my family that I was going to medical school, my parents and aunts and uncles went bananas! I sometimes wonder, even now, if I didn't become a doctor because that was what my parents expected. You know my dad was called a "healing doc" by the farming community we lived in. He even got paid sometimes with eggs and slabs of bacon. He never complained. When I first listened to what you had to say with the spiral, I thought immediately of my dad. He literally lived a personal and professional life that was directed by his soul. That must have been the reason that there seemed to be great meaning for him no matter what he did – even in so many of the little things he was called upon to do in his medical practice.

Bill: I couldn't help but notice how comfortably you used the word soul as you spoke about your experience of your father.

Pete: That's true! Ever since "Medicine in Search of Meaning" I couldn't get that spiral out of my mind. I even talked about it with my wife – about the higher self, the soul, the spiritual core of power and energy with which we are born. I've been thinking a lot these days about what really matters to me. And do you know what it is? To stay more consciously aware and connected to the real source of power in my life because it will help me be an even better doctor, father and husband.

Bill: And how do you choose to do that?

Pete: Several things are beginning to change both in my practice of medicine and in my home life. I've decided to spend time – about 10 to 15 minutes each day that I'm working in the clinic or making rounds – in quiet reflection. Just thinking about why I'm doing what I'm doing and about why I became a physician in the first place ... things like that. Not forcing answers to come ... just being still ... kind of getting off the treadmill that I have been complaining about for years. Medical journals are not the only things I read now. Novels and biographies that inspire me are becoming part of my reading diet. Also, and I haven't told a lot of folks this, religious studies are becoming one of my favorite subjects. Sometimes I daydream and think about a life apart from medicine and see myself teaching at a university. Does that sound crazy or what? I'm learning to say no to some things in my professional life – like committee involvement, some speaking engagements and the like. I want to be part of my kids' life. I guess you could say I'm creating a little more balance in my life. I probably will never leave medicine, but I can still dream, can't I?

Pete was not the exception to the hundreds of physicians I have worked with over the past several years. Those with whom I have been able to talk in some depth have shared, in one way or another, that the biggest challenge they face as physicians is to create a sense of balance in their personal and professional lives – to break out of the mold that medical training seems to favor. I have shared with them – as I often reflect upon myself – that every decision we make, every action we take, either moves us closer to identifying with our personality/ego (all those areas on the outer arcs of the spiral) or with our soul, the primary source of empowerment that gives meaning and purpose to life. This is the change – using my words, not theirs – that I see happening ever so slowly, ever so quietly, within the physician world that I am encountering.

Self Reflection: For the sake of balance

How do you learn to choose to live out of authentic power when you have been and are part of a system that ignores the spiritual dimension of physicians' lives? Are you bringing all of you into you practice of medicine, into your examining room, into your patients' hospital room – or just your diagnostic skills, knowledge base and/or technological expertise, as important as they are? What are you leaving in your car as you step each day into the world of medicine? Why, in fact, are you on this earth doing medicine and not something else? (Or, what is your motivation for continuing to practice medicine? Does anything need to change?) Where indeed is your source of power or identity beyond pills and scalpels, IV tubes and X-rays? What would your life be like if you were fully engaged in it, with a quality balance, as a clinician, a lover, a father/mother, etc.? How are you contributing to a culture in medicine that values caring as well as curing, where death is not the enemy but a rite of passage, that equally values and gives credence to rational, scientific thought as it does to intuitive, creative reflection? If we don't know where we are going, any direction will do.

Your thoughts along the way

*(Take a moment to write down any thoughts
or insights you want to remember.)*

Case Studies and Reflection

Have you ever been in a situation where you were afraid of making the "right" decision because of a misplaced sense of loyalty or fear of offending someone? If so, these samplings of various case studies might be thought provoking.

Case Studies

Dr. Jack P. knows that a colleague of his, a 69-year-old OB/GYN, is losing her skill level, especially in the delivery room. She doesn't make split second decisions like she used to. Jack also observes this OB/GYN having memory lapses. The OB/GYN stubbornly refuses to talk about retirement. During a recent delivery, the baby's heart rate shows deceleration patterns on the monitor. She does not perform a C-section and the baby is stillborn. Jack learns about this and does nothing.

Dr. Sharon S. is a second-year family practice resident. One of the doctors who does teaching rounds with the residents has made sexual advances to Sharon on three separate occasions. Sharon is afraid to say anything to anyone for fear she would get into trouble. She rationalizes to herself: "This is just the good old boys at work and play." She does nothing and says nothing to anyone.

Dr. Pete P. has discovered that one of his clinic colleagues is manipulating her Medicare billings – billing for services that are not being performed. He has proof of this doctor's fraudulent activity, but decides not to do anything. He just buries his head in the sand and pretends that it will go away. Pete is afraid of what other physicians might say about his uncovering "one of their own."

Self-Reflection

"Spinach/Popeye/Medicine" …a cure for what ails ya!

When Popeye needed courage and strength in difficult situations, he opened a can of spinach and gulped it down. Presto! Magically, he would be transformed into a superhuman, capable of dealing with his arch nemesis Brutus. He would save Olive Oyl and all was right with Popeye's world!

Several key questions emerge for me whenever I think about my own courage, power or strength. I offer them to you. Where is your "can of spinach" when confronted with difficult experiences? Where do you look and what is it you want to access when you look there? Especially in your interactions with your peers: Where is your source of power and how do you access it when the truth is needed in a given situation? What helps you overcome the fears, the rationalizations and the excuses for not acting and communicating in demanding situations? In these defining moments (opportunities for new growth and insight) does your power to speak diminish because of the power you have turned over to others? Reread the three samplings of case studies again with these questions in the forefront of your mind.

Your spiritual center is your can of spinach.
Spirituality and the spiritual journey can be described as the process of recognizing and growing into a power or energy that we are born with – a power/energy that when accessed impels us towards wholeness and new life. It is the power at the center of who we are (our spiritual center) that can be our can of spinach. Our ego, our mind, can play tricks on us when we look to it for strength in difficult relational situations. It can easily let us down. Consciously connecting to our deepest self (soul) enables us to speak the truth. To access our inner power we must hold our life still and reflect on the question: "What is this experience asking of me?" It means waiting for an answer beyond what our mind can offer initially.

You can change your thinking.
Granted - confrontation is hard, downright difficult at times. It is especially hard to confront a colleague. I suggest that what makes it hard is the way we think about it. If we label it as disloyalty, selling out, or rocking the boat, then it will be that for us. If we think about speaking the truth as an opportunity for caring, for enhancing the

good of others and ultimately as an opportunity to extend friendship and mutual respect, the encounter with a colleague takes on a different perspective. Our perspective is, as always, our choice to make.

Your medical practice includes your colleagues.
Medical school training does not teach physicians to access their spiritual power and use it within the context of professional relationships. Sometimes the practice of medicine demands that physicians view their practices to include not only their patients, but also their responsibilities to their colleagues.

Your attention is power.
"I give power to that which I pay attention" is applicable here. If we allow feelings and thoughts of intimidation, fear and anxiety to prevail in our imagination, we give them power over ourselves. If, on the other hand, we locate the internal source of our power (and therefore meaning and purpose) and pay conscious attention to its dynamic, we will allow that power to guide our decision-making and actions. Again, the choice is ours. The capacity to practice medicine is more than scientific knowledge, technological application and skill development. It includes a conscious connection to the real source of physician power – our spiritual center.

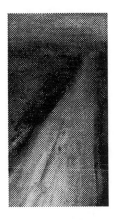

Chapter Four

POPEYE, SPINACH, AND RELATIONAL POWER

There are at least two mysteries of the universe that I know nothing about. I have been perplexed since childhood. One centers around my imagination: what was in the closet that got me laughing every time Fibber opened it on the old radio show Fibber McGee and Molly? The other one focuses on this deeply philosophic question: How in the hell did Popeye open his can of spinach? Did you ever seen him use a can opener? Not I! Yet, when he needed strength and power to beat up on his arch nemesis, Brutus, the can of spinach magically opened. You know the rest – Olive Oyl was saved, Brutus was beaten, and Popeye could be heard muttering: "I am what I am and that's all that I am!" The End.

Both Fibber McGee and Popeye knew something profound. The power for both laughter and physical strength is on the inside. Whenever a laugh was needed, I just knew the closet door would open. The rest was left up to my imagination. Whenever Popeye was in trouble, it was what was inside the can of spinach that gave strength and courage. In much the same way as these two examples afford, it is what is inside of us that determine how we express power, how we experience and cultivate it. Unlike my two old-time examples, I will be describing what is in the "closet" of power as well as how to find and use an opener for the "spinach."

Expressions of power

Before I even begin presenting these ideas, let me say clearly: both relational and unilateral expressions of power are needed. One is not better than the other, per se. As I will discuss later, it is precisely the situation in which we find ourselves at any given moment that determines an appropriate response in terms of our behavior and attitude. The real issue, then, is the question of orientation. What is our basic and fundamental orientation in terms of exercising power? Are we oriented more towards one form or the other?

Relational power can best be described as the capacity to nurture and sustain personal/professional relationships. It is the experience of power that truly respects and honors the other. Relationally powerful people have the ability to produce an effect and to receive one as well; to be affected as well as to affect, to be influenced as well as to influence. Essentially, in the human exchange and encounter, power becomes a shared experience, a two-way street, that imbues each person with increased stature and respect, rather than depleting one so the other can expand. Relational expressions of power never diminish life. Each person in the encounter is validated. The dynamics of a relationally powerful experience can be seen metaphorically by using an image of a "two-way street". Two cars approach each other from different directions, each having its own space on the street. One car's direction is not more important than the other. Whether one car is a Mercedes Benz and the other a Chevrolet makes no difference. Each is what it is. As long as each car stays in its own lane and does not try to take more space on the road than allocated to it, the encounter is smooth as they pass. Each car and driver respects its own space and in so doing, respects the space of the other car and driver. Both will reach their appointed destinations without doing violence. Accidents happen when one car wants to control the entire road – or the portion of the road allotted to the other.

The opposite of relational power is unilateral power. The chief characteristic of unilateral power is the capacity to produce an effect, to exert an influence, to affect the other. Its major trait is control. The unilaterally powerful person seeks power over others to enhance the self. Whenever we operate out of a unilateral expression of power, our value increases at the expense of the other. Our stature, at least in our own eyes and possibly in the eyes of others, becomes determined by our ability to control the external situation, that is, having power over the environment, over others, and over events. This is how we measure success in life – by our acquisitions, our posturing, our winning the argument, our beating the other competitively, etc. Our personal power portfolio is enhanced, and hence our life is enhanced, to the degree that we have control over our experiences and the external world around us. Competition and fear are major players in a unilaterally powerful person's life. Fear of losing and of not being the best in a given field of endeavor are prime motivators for the unilaterally oriented person. Failure is a character defect, not an opportunity to learn and change. Using the metaphor of the road again: unilaterally oriented drivers want the whole road to themselves. Instead of respecting life as a two-way street – each car respecting the space of the other (mutuality) – the unilateral driver wants the whole enchilada, with little or no respect or honor for the space of other cars. Our focus is narrow – get to the desired destination no matter whom we have to run over! We control the road and everyone else better look out for us. Here we come! The typical "climbing the corporate ladder" is one expression of unilateral power. For us to get to where we want to go is key even if that means stepping on others on the way up. Unilaterally oriented people live in a world of winners and losers.

There are some behavior patterns that are characteristic of both orientations of power. Imagine a spectrum from 1 to 10: 1 being the purest expression of relational power and 10 being the purest expression of unilateral power (see fig.4:1). Few, if any of us, would be a pure 1 or a pure 10. But based on our habitual patterns of behavior over time, we develop an orientation and land somewhere on that spectrum. As you reflect on the various behaviors and attitudes on the chart, locate where your basic orientation might be.

The Power Spectrum

Relational Power	Unilateral Power
the capacity to nurture and sustain personal/professional relationships	the capacity to influence others (one dimensional)

```
|  1                            5                            10  |
|                                                                |
```

__1. Power with others	__1. Power over others
__2. Responsible with others (collaboration)	__2. Responsible with others (hierarchical)
__3. Giving and receiving	__3. Giving only
__4. Mobility (space to grow)	__4. Bound and restrictive
__5. Teamwork (connectedness)	__5. Individuality (separateness)
__6. Empowering	__6. Controlling
__7. Feelings expressed	__7. Feelings repressed or hidden
__8. Balance between content and process	__8. Content oriented
__9. "I learn from others too!" (two-way street)	__9. "Others learn from me!" (one-way street)
__10. Flexibility	__10. Rigidity
__11. Self worth grounded inside	__11. Self worth grounded in productivity

Figure 4:1

Physicians and unilateral power

Physicians are taught to become unilaterally powerful. Is that causing problems?

Spirituality is at its very roots a journey into relational power. It is not dependent on what we own, the degrees we have or do not have, the social status we have achieved or not achieved, or hundreds of other things external and tangential to who we are internally.

In the established world of medical science, and specifically in the training of medical students, there is a great myth created and taught that is causing tremendous tension and anxiety in the lives of practitioners today. Success as a physician is often measured by how well this myth is carried out. The myth is exacerbated by the very people medicine serves. Our culture expects the myth to achieve its outcomes. The myth is not taught directly, even consciously. But it is all pervasive in the clinical practice of medicine today. Here is the myth in a nutshell: "Science is god and as god I have the answers. Learn of me, but have no false gods before me. Give homage to me and I will give you dominion over the physical world."

In other words, the power of physicians is enhanced in direct proportion to their capacity to unilaterally affect their patients; to have power over their patients' diseases via knowledge, skill development and diagnostic ability; and to carry around inside of themselves the subtle (and sometimes not so subtle) belief that they know what is best.

In this mythological world, however, tensions are created and anxieties are raised for the physician. Death is seen as the enemy, diseases are seen as diagnostic challenges, and the patient gets somehow abstracted from the doctor/patient relationship. In most cases, none of this is done on a conscious, deliberative level. Physicians have told me that this "god of science" myth has been ingrained in them since medical school. As one 62-year-old surgeon so abruptly put it to me: "People put us on high perches – expecting us to perform as gods. My problem is that I bought into that fallacy without even knowing it!" A young resident shared this with me: "Medical schools and residency programs are threatened by anything that can't be put under a micro-scope and examined. Spirituality is a threat because you can't see or touch it directly; therefore, does it exist?"

Now I am not suggesting in the least that physicians slack off in their understanding of medical science and the best that it has to offer. I certainly would want the very best surgeon if I needed surgery. What I am suggesting very strongly, however, is the concern I hear from some physicians that there is more to practicing medicine than simply applying medical science in given cases. The "more" I am referring to is integrating the human, spiritual side of physician development into the medical model that so characterizes the practice of medicine today. In point of fact, I believe, physician's practices can be enhanced through this integration.

Debunking the myth

Physicians learn from patients.

Physicians are problem solvers to a large extent. A patient comes with a problem, a diagnosis is made, and an appropriate resolution to the problem is offered. Next case. This pattern goes on and on, each case perhaps offering some new wrinkle. People feel terrible and want to get fixed. That is why they come to physicians, because physicians have something that is needed. Relationally powerful physicians, in addition to bringing their skills and diagnostic capacities into the examining room, will also allow themselves to be open to learning from their patients. Patients, too, have something to offer. This mindset is very different from what is taught in medical school. What patients have to offer is this: the opportunity for a physician to learn how to be a better physician, primarily on the human side of the equation. A relationally powerful physician has developed an attitude, a belief, that with each patient encounter, there is an opportunity for growth. A belief in the equality of being can be generated and nourished. What is brought to the table, in other words, is an attitude on the physicians' part that rec-ognizes why patients come to their physicians in the first place, but also recognizes and consciously accepts that the physician is also involved in receiving something from the encounter. Physicians have something to gain precisely because they are investing more than just medical, scientific knowledge into the physician/patient relationship. When this happens, the patient is never abstracted from the process. In fact, patients in this scenario empower physicians and become their primary teachers. More than simply practicing medicine goes on in the examining room.

You bring your relationship with soul to your patients.
As the above belief system begins to take hold in physicians' consciousness, then a certain dynamic can evolve which I call "clearing a path to the soul." If our response to the "who am I?" question goes beyond identifying solely with what we do, then it makes sense to ask this question: "What am I doing to nurture a relationship with my own inner spirit, my soul?" Not to respond to this question affirmatively would be like asking a friend for help when we haven't done anything to cultivate the relationship for several years. It could be hard opening the door again. One of the ways of thinking about relational power is to speak of our soul and the power of our soul. Our soul loves life in every form that it appears, does not judge an experience (or a person) as good or bad, and sees meaning and purpose in even the smallest details of everyday life. As I bring these thoughts to consciousness and translate them into purposeful activity, a relationship (a friendship) is developed with the energy of my soul. The very experience of that dynamic is what a physician can bring into the examining room or to the hospital bedside.

As your soul is enhanced, so is the soul of another.
This power of the soul, a relationally powerful force in our life, is contrasted with the power of ego or personality, which is by and large unilaterally oriented. One indication that we are clearing the path to our soul is when we align our thoughts, feelings and behaviors with the highest and deepest part of ourselves. Life, then, has a real chance to become rich and full. Fears dissolve and the drive of our ego to control all aspects of our life diminishes. Spiritually rooted physicians, for example, have learned to develop a keen awareness that their power lies not only in their medical acumen, but also in the nourishing and developing of their soul power in action. Truly empowered physicians are ones who literally are incapable of using others to achieve ends or desired goals. Rather, they see in their own lives and the lives of others

as parallel universes unfolding – as our universe, our person, our soul is enhanced, so is the universe, the person, the soul of the other. For physicians, "the other" could be colleagues, patients, family and anyone else who is part of their universe.

Although roles are different, there is equality of being.
In the world of medicine – a world of diagnoses, technological applications, drugs, insurance forms, peer review committees, and the like – relationally powerful physicians begin to see that through human interactions a dynamic energy or synergy develops that acts like a magnet which draws to the soul of each participant a new awareness that there is equality of being in the human family, but different roles or functions that are performed for the good of all. This awareness is not grounded in the roles performed but in the souls of each performer.

Experience is a means for growth.
The souls of relationally powerful physicians see each experience in life as yet another opportunity to explode the myth of the god of science as all pervasive. Pain and suffering become birthplaces for creative insight for both physician and patient. Experiences are neither good nor bad; they are simply lessons our souls and egos have been given to clear a straighter pathway to deeper meaning and purpose in the clinical practice of medicine and beyond. Especially during these crazy times in the world of health care, physicians see more clearly now that their souls need the sometimes stormy waters of experience in order to grow. A different context is created for practicing medicine – one that has traded in total control and a "we've always done it this way" attitude for acceptance, receptivity to change, and a willingness to keep on learning.

A case study in futility
"You alone can do it, but you can't do it alone!"

"I don't give a damn what the insurance company says, I want another ultrasound for my patient – and I want it approved today! Don't take any crap from those folks!" So began another typical day for Judy P., an OB/GYN who is in a group practice with two other physicians. Judy is 42 years old, divorced, and has two children, ages 7 and

9, living at home with her. The demands of her practice have been overwhelming for several years, consistently causing her life to become unbalanced. Anger and resentment over a failed marriage and a messy divorce have left Judy in a state of fury that has been brought into the clinic and her practice. She is increasingly becoming snappy at nurses and office staff and literally blows off steam when dealing with insurance companies. Her clinic partners walk on egg shells around her, dreading to ask her to cover for them at unscheduled times. Recently having settled out of court on a malpractice suit, Judy continues to blame this misfortune on her ex-husband. Seeing little of her children except on weekends, Judy has deep feelings of guilt about her role as mother. However, up until now, she was able to avoid those feelings by plunging into her practice. She has even considered leaving medicine and getting an MBA. A plaque on her wall said: "You alone can do it, but you can't do it alone!"

I often question myself like this: Why do I allow my life to get so out of whack? Shouldn't I know better? Aren't I smart enough not to get so off balance that I feel distressed and miserable in some areas of my life? Why do I allow the behaviors and attitudes of others to throw me off track so that I become angry and resentful? Aren't I mature enough not to let outside influences bother me? Is my happiness and joy so dependent on people being the kind of people I want them to be that I am now enslaved when they aren't? (I kind of like that last question!)

The futility that Judy is experiencing in her life is largely brought on by her choices, often not conscious ones at that. For her, medicine is a safe familiar home – a profession where she literally can lose herself whenever things don't go her way. Plunging into her practice, keeping up with her reading, and going to medical conferences that are meant to enhance her professional skill and knowledge base, have left Judy still feeling miserable when she is alone and not doing something or other. What is the answer for Judy – or for each of us – when we feel out of sorts, when our lives get out of balance, when what we most want (love, meaning and acceptance) is not there for long stretches? The answer can be found in believing and acting out of a belief in this statement: "You alone can do it, but you can't do it alone!"

Creating balance

So much of a physician's identity is tied up with knowledge, science, skill development and the general feeling of "at homeness" with practicing medicine. As I interviewed physicians and observed them in action, I began to see that, like Judy, they can easily forget about developing their own soul life, their own spiritual life. The doctor persona is a powerful, positive gift that is projected out into the community. A doctor's soul life needs to be projected out into the community and with patients as well, in alignment with scientific skills and knowledge. When there is balance, when quality time and mindfulness are spent in both cultivating the art of soul development along with the art of being a doctor, then, it seems to me, alignment happens. With that alignment comes deeper meaning and purpose for the individual physician.

There are two key ideas that can assist us in creating balance: 1) an understanding of how power and energy are cultivated; and 2) how to be mindful of caring for ourselves. Power and energy are experienced and cultivated in two distinct ways: relationally or unilaterally. The relational experience of power is the capacity to both produce an effect as well as to receive one, a giving and a receiving. Essentially, it is characterized as a two-way street. Unilateral power is the capacity to produce an effect only, a giving only, a one-way street. Relationally powerful growth is enhanced by both giving and receiving. Physicians will grow by both giving from their knowledge and skill base as well as being open to the lessons that life offers. Unilaterally powerful people (like Judy) deplete their energy levels because they believe they are somebody (identity) because of what they can do for others. There is very little receptivity to change for unilaterally powerful people.

Mindfulness, that is, the capacity to focus energy and attention, on the total person that makes us who we are is a key ingredient in growth. Physicians who learn that there is a soul deep inside that needs to be cared for like a beautiful rose garden will be more able to bring their skills as physicians into alignment with some of the deeper realities of that soul.

Self-Reflection

How do you take care of the person behind the diagnostic skills, behind the practitioner of medicine? How can you be open to the influences of others, i.e., family, friends, colleagues, patients, etc.? What are the lessons you need to learn in your life right now? What is your life asking of you – and what are you asking of your life? Have you been trying to cultivate a lifestyle that doesn't require your presence? (I really like that question!)

"Come to the edge!" "No, we will fall."

"Come to the edge!" "No, we will fall."

They came to the edge. They were pushed. And they flew.

Your Thoughts Along The Way

(Take a moment to write down any thoughts
or insights you want to remember.)

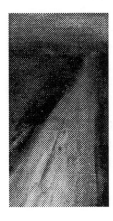

Chapter Five

FEAR OF CHANGE

"Insanity is doing the same things over and over again and expecting a different result!"

I had an occasion to travel to Washington D.C. recently. Sandwiched in between my visits to the congressional delegation from Wisconsin, I took time to roam around the Capitol Hill area. I just wandered, with no particular place to go. Now I am a great believer that some of the most creative times of my life are the so called "in between" times when my mind is on hold and all agendas cease. During those times, my creative energies are not focused on a project or other purposeful activity, and are allowed to come and go at will. As I passed a book store, I noticed a poster of the Lincoln Memorial with the following thought from Abraham Lincoln printed on the bottom: "If we know where we are, and perhaps a bit about how we got there, we might be able to see where we are tending, and thereby affect our destiny." Lincoln's thought stayed with me for some time. It made such an impression on me that it still enters my consciousness at other "in between" times in my life. Sometimes it even surfaces in the context of talking with others. One such time occurred during an interview with Pamela, an obstetrician/gynecologist who practices in an urban area of Wisconsin. Pamela and I were nearly an hour into our planned two-hour session when I began to notice some large doses of resistance whenever the subject of change came up. Here is part of that interview.

Pamela: You asked me what I liked most about my medical training. I haven't thought about it for a while, but... I guess it was the fact that everything seemed predictable to me. That's the word – predictable. Each and every course I took had specific goals and objectives that I could see were applicable to my future as a physician. The course lectures were well organized, the lab experiments were actually fun for me... you know, using my hands and translating my knowledge through the use of my hands. I always knew what to expect if I followed directions, learned the formulas correctly, and listened to my teachers. Even exams had a certain appeal to me. I knew that by memorizing some things and being able to conceptualize in logical sequence other things, I would do well. I learned to rely on myself. I learned that if I did what I knew I could do, I could control the outcome. That's why I loved science so much – I could measure it, study it and have predictable outcomes.

Bill: You spoke about predictability and control and alluded to science as a way of offering that to you. Could you say more about this in terms of your current practice of medicine?

Pamela: Okay, but I would need to start back around 1980 or so when I was accepted into a multi-specialty clinic and began practicing medicine. I was a product of the sixties and seventies but only tangentially. You see, while some of my classmates who weren't in premed were involved in the anti-war movement and other social causes of the day, I was hunkered down in a dorm room studying. I insulated myself from the cultural revolution that was happening all around me and for just reason – studies were my priority and good grades my quest. Nothing else seemed to matter at the time. The more I saw of the Kent State type of experiences and the race riots in large urban areas, the more I plunged into my studies. I was afraid, I think, and I don't really know why. Well, anyway, I simply never did well with change. My only close friends were in medical school – isolated like I was. In 1980 when I hung up my shingle, life was sweet and uncomplicated. The long hours were an exciting challenge. Medicine was my life and it was what I knew best. I'd make my rounds, deliver babies, and see patients in my office. For me, these years up to 1989 were the golden ones.

Bill: Why was that the case for you?

Pamela: I loved what I was doing, getting paid handsomely for doing *it, and I met the man I eventually married in 1986. It was a happy time for me. I was all about doing what I dreamed about doing. As my dad used to say, "I was on schedule." My son Christopher was born in 1988. I never had to pay attention to the growing number of changes that were happening out there in the health care field – mergers, the buying up of physician practices and the like. My accountant paid my bills and kept me informed on how I was doing. Every once in awhile I went to hospital sponsored meetings to learn about these changes and how they impacted me; but nothing honestly made an impression. What woke me up occurred in late 1989 when I got a call from some young puppy from a utilization review department in one of the insurance HMOs in which I was participating. He informed me that I was not authorized to deliver a multiple birth pregnancy at the hospital I wanted. I had to go to one across town – one that didn't have a neonatal intensive care unit. I was livid! This kind of crap had happened before, but for some reason I reacted strongly. How could an insurance company tell me how and where to practice medicine. That was only the start of things to come. Bottom line: I was fearful that I was losing my independence and ability to practice medicine on my terms.*

Bill: It sounds to me like you could no longer insulate yourself emotionally from the changes that were occurring around you, especially in the health care arena. Maybe the days of stay in your dorm room and ignoring the world around you were over?

Pamela: That's right! And I'm damn angry about it too. Health care reform, or more aptly socialized medicine, integrated delivery systems, buying up physician practices like mine – it's all bullshit! If it's not broke, don't fix it! I was doing just fine until the lawyers and politicians entered the picture. I get angry more now than I ever used to. Even one of my colleagues told me to slow down and smell the roses. My marriage broke up in early '93. I guess I can't blame Carl. Why is this happening to me? What did I ever do to deserve this? I am a damn good physician, Bill. Why me?

Pamela's capacity to deal with change was fairly typical of the many physicians with whom I have worked and have come to know over the years. I have experienced physicians to be very focused people who are called upon to make often split-second decisions on their feet. That is their gift to their patients. It is a result of living in a very structured learning environment that is, in fact, predictable. A+B=C. If you have these symptoms plus these symptoms, then you must have this or that illness. The structured world of science is predictable.

What I have found, however, is the shadow side to the capacity to focus and make decisions in the structured world of science. The shadow side includes the inability to create and be open to more expansive and non-scientific ways of thinking (mental constructs) about reality – especially the reality that characterizes the world of today's medical system and service delivery. The challenge of being open to a different way of thinking about "life as a physician in the practice of medicine," often falls by the wayside. The pull is so strong to stay in the safe haven of "what we know works" – a way of thinking that rewards the faithful and causes discomfort for those who would question the established world of medicine.

One physician expressed it this way: "I was trained in an either...or world, not a both...and one. To me, that means I better stay focused on what the medical establishment has defined for me on the question of 'what makes a good doctor?' To break the mold is implicitly frowned upon. For example, there is an unwritten code that says always back up one of your own. I know a doc that makes mistake after mistake, most recently one of his mistakes causing severe problems for a newborn. Others docs covered for him. I was so irate when I heard what happened that I went up to him and demanded he give up practicing medicine, at least until he could develop new skills."

A neurologist told me that on occasion he refers some of his pain management patients to a Rolfer (rolfing being a form of deep body work called structural integration). One of his partners heard about this and told him to never let the word out about what he was doing. His reason: referrals would dry up because he would be labeled a "new ager." Change is happening all around health care these days – internally in terms of the ongoing rapid growth of medical science and technology, and externally in terms of new business affiliations and political agendas. The whitewater rapids of change are here. Many

physicians are paddling up stream simply because they have great difficulty in dealing with change and find it far easier to resist it. Advances
in medical science are easily accepted. What is not so easy to accept are
changes to the image of what a physician should be in the world
according to the traditional medical establishment. The human, spiritual dimension gets lost in the shuffle, as do the emotions, personal
relationships, and most everything else outside the world of medicine.
Change is resisted in these areas, as a physician once told me, precisely
because "all we were taught was the science of medicine." She went on
to add: "We were engaged in a myopic view of the world – a world
that causes discomfort. Like children running to mom, we could
always retreat to the bosom of medicine to get our bearings straight!
Therein was not only our refuge and our strength, but this mother
held our identity maternally in her hands."

The nature of change and the evolution of meaning

Following is depiction of the cyclical nature of change and the
evolving of new meaning.

How, then, can we deal with change and see it as an ally rather
than a threat? How do we participate in it as ally, and in so doing
derive greater meaning and purpose in our clinical practice of medicine? This is the question that I would like to unpack for the purposes
of offering a different mental construct for physicians (and all of us) to
consciously consider. The challenging issue as we go through this exer-
cise together is rooted in the belief that we cannot change anyone, we
can only change ourselves. As we change our attitude, behaviors, and
belief systems, we will create an environment that invites others to
change too.

This diagram (see fig.5:1), uses a bell curve to portray an individual's developmental growth curve. The upward arc represents the generative side of our life cycle as we respond to issues and situations
involving change and the discovery of meaning. The downward arc
represents the degenerative side to our life cycle as we resist change. At
the outset, I am suggesting that we discover meaning and purpose only
when we are living on the generative side of the curve. The degenera-

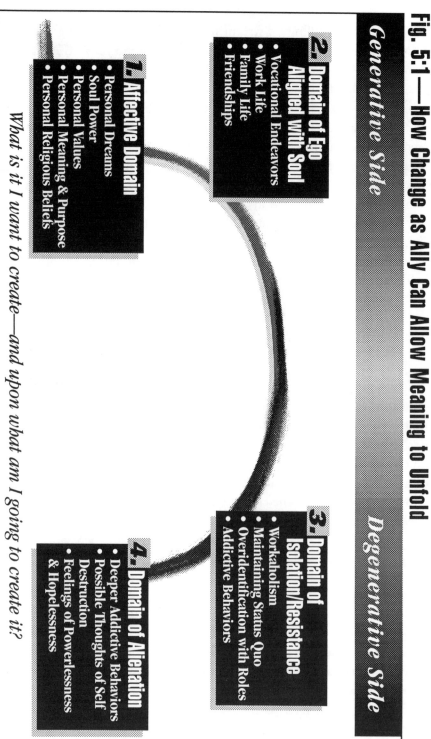

Fig. 5:1—How Change as Ally Can Allow Meaning to Unfold

Generative Side

Degenerative Side

2. Domain of Ego Aligned with Soul
- Vocational Endeavors
- Work Life
- Family Life
- Friendships

1. Affective Domain
- Personal Dreams
- Soul Power
- Personal Values
- Personal Meaning & Purpose
- Personal Religious Beliefs

3. Domain of Isolation/Resistance
- Workaholism
- Maintaining Status Quo
- Overidentification with Roles
- Addictive Behaviors

4. Domain of Alienation
- Deeper Addictive Behaviors
- Possible Thoughts of Self Destruction
- Feelings of Powerlessness & Hopelessness

What is it I want to create—and upon what am I going to create it?

world that they are happy and find meaning in their work.

One such unhappy camper was a physician with whom I spoke several years ago. She had been in private practice for over ten years and shared this with me: "I am living proof that a person cannot live out the dreams of her parents. It was always their dream that I become a doctor. They recently died and so has their dream. I will be leaving medicine soon – going back to school to become the teacher that I always wanted to be. I guess I am finally finding my path after being on theirs for so long." For this woman to change, she needed to return to quadrant #1 and reclaim her dream. Her new quadrant #2 activity will now be aligned with her quadrant #1.

One of the most wonderful and magnificent questions that quadrant #2 can offer is this: "What is it that we want to create in our life (quadrant #2 activity) and upon what will we create it (quadrant #1 activity)?" This question is not only important for quadrant #2 experiences, but it will become the bridge question that enables us to reconnect with meaning and purpose when we find myself mired in quadrant #3, the degenerative side to our lived experience. There is a beautiful metaphor that I often use to describe the relationship between the quadrants: quadrant #1 becomes the navigating force from within (our internal radar), guiding us through the events and experiences of our life and the choices we make. In times of chaos – times of rapid change – we can access that power and energy to guide and touch whatever we do. This navigating force is always available to us no matter where we find ourselves. No one can ever take it away nor diminish its power.

Whenever we experience ourselves living out of the energy generated in quadrant #2, it is a sure bet that we are aligned with our soul even though we may not always be conscious of this happening. We will have developed a heightened sense of being relationally present to others and to our work life, thus affording us the opportunity to feel more deeply that meaning and purpose are major players in our life. This will happen no matter what situations our life presents. Even pain and suffering have a chance to become birthplaces for creative insight. The varied experiences of our life are but a continuum of lessons to be learned and as such are neither good nor bad – they simply are. We may feel rage, anger, hurt or disappointment, but we will have learned to give ourselves some "alone time" or "quiet time" to reflect on the experience, to own it as ours, and to use it as our teacher. We are exactly where we need to be in our life – regardless of what is happening to us or around us. For example, physicians grounded in quadrant #2 living will begin to view their patients as teachers that will indeed teach them how to be better, more compassionate and empathetic physicians. Even those patients who were a pain to see and a source of aggravation are now transformed in the mind of a physician to a teacher, not pain in the posterior! Patients become gifts from which to grow, not sources of grief to complain about or avoid.

Isolation, loss of control, and resistance (Quadrant #3)

Refer back to figure 5:1 and notice the top of the curve where the WE/I is located. The doorway to moving into the degenerative side of our life's journey begins with the loss of a sense of "we-ness", that is, not recognizing and living out of a relational power base. The journey into the degenerative side continues in the various ways we learn to isolate ourselves from others – a kind of numbing process that can eventually take on addictive proportions. A general feeling of powerlessness wedges itself into our mind set and we allow ourselves, not always in a conscious way, to become a victim in our world. Oftentimes, this victimization occurs in times of change when we feel that our life is out of control, when new things happen and challenge us to respond. Instead of responding, we react to the changing environment using the tools of anger, blame, rationalization and even self-pity.

Even though we may not be aware of what is really happening to us, there is a growing and deepening sense of discontent and discomfort. Change becomes our biggest foe because we feel we are losing our anchor, that is, our ability to control the situation and make it more comfortable for us in which to function.

A sure sign of the experience of quadrant #3 living is feeling out of control and experiencing a loss of predictability coupled with the paradoxical situation of trying to regain control through ego enhancement via unilateral power behaviors. The sad and often troubling part of being locked in the degenerative side of our life's journey rests in the fact that we truly believe the answer to all of our life's problems rests in the very thing that got us to where I am – trying to control the people and events in our life to meet our expectations of what should or should not be. The following case study illustrates this point very clearly.

A case study on victim mentality

James U. is a 52-year-old cardiologist practicing in a town of 60,000 people. He is one of three cardiologists in the area. Because of all the changes in payment for and delivery of health care services, James is being "squeezed out of the market" (his own words) by primary care doctors who are doing more and more primary cardiology. Even some of the non-emergency acute cardiac patients are being referred to major medical centers. HMOs and other managed care insurance payors are not allowing referrals to James as they used to. He has turned into a very angry physician, blaming every one from politicians to the insurance industry to the Catholic sisters who sponsor the hospital for his plight. During medical staff meetings, James is the "bitcher and moaner" who is so negative about everything that his colleagues do not like being around him. "I am a victim of that liberal crowd that wants to change health care. Even these nuns are trying to take away my livelihood by all this merger and acquisition talk. I've been damn loyal to this hospital and to the community. All I get in return is a pile of shit for thanks!"

What was sad is that James could not see that he has choices, that he has the internal power and energy to respond creatively to the situations of change that were befalling his life. He uses blame and intense anger as weapons of choice to deal with his experiences. I asked him a quadrant #1 question: "What in you needs to change in order to meaningfully continue practicing medicine now and into the future?" I might as well have spoken in Chinese for all James cared. He simply could not get underneath the dark side of his ego and entertain this question in a reflective manner.

Pamela (the OB/GYN from the beginning of this chapter) was also grounded in quadrant #3 living all through medical school and on into the first several years of her practice. For many people like Pamela and James, it will often take a huge, sometimes catastrophic, experience to call attention that something needs to change – and more importantly, that something is available to us, namely quadrant #1 activity. For Pamela, the divorce from her husband shocked her into getting assistance to deal with and work through the challenges of change in her life. For James, it might be the loss of medical staff privileges or simply a dried up marketplace for his services. For others, addictive behaviors like alcoholism, over-eating or compulsive gambling might bring the person to a crisis point in life. Resistance to change is especially strong for quadrant #3 physicians. Their training does little or nothing to orient them towards meaningful quadrant #1 and #2 activity.

Whatever our particular set of circumstances that ground us in quadrant #3 living for a time, increased activity and a more determined task orientation (the underlying belief being: the more we do, the faster we'll get out of this mess!) will leave little if any room for reflection. Balance gets tossed out of the window and is replaced by a unilateral quest to put our life together – no matter what the cost, no matter over whom we have to step to do it. What occurs, then, is a widening of the gulf between our ego and our soul – our soul going to a very quiet place inside and our ego assuming a dominant role. For physicians, this can result in a loss of the human side of their clinical practice and hence a further denial of the dream that led them into medicine in the first place.

Another aspect of this degenerative side – and one that more deeply grounds us into the resistance trap – is characterized by a growing sense of powerlessness and imbalance in our life. Powerlessness comes from seeing ourselves as being a victim to the changes going on all around us. For physicians this might take the form of the new health care management or payment methods, the acquisition of physician practices, increased paperwork and regulations, and the hundred and one other ways the field of medical practice has changed so dramatically over the past few years. Even the public perception of doctors is changing from one of "being on a pedestal" to "make a mistake and I'll call my lawyer." (One physician told me privately that he would "like to stay God-like and perfect in the eyes of the public for a while longer" because "my patients are not ready to see the real me, with all my faults and failings.")

As our life gets more and more out of balance, those closest to us – family, friends and even colleagues – bear the brunt of our lack of awareness. Less and less time is spent with family, especially our spouse. Working late and long hours, volunteering to be on every medical committee that comes our way, taking on more and more patients – become byproducts of our imbalanced life. If the truth be told, many physicians have told me that "this is just the way it is. Don't you know that I am doing all of this because I love my family and want to better their life?" A great rationalization for remaining in a workaholic mode! When I asked the physicians who responded in this way to describe their relationship with their spouse, universally, each of them said something along these lines: "Things were not real good – a lot of tension in the family that my spouse blames me for. He/she is always on my case. No wonder I work so hard! It's one thing to hear the complaints of my patients – it's another to hear it from my spouse."

Whatever it is in our life that causes it to be imbalanced, this truism hits the mark: When we are faced with a distressful situation, our tendency to return to a place of comfort for relief is strong. The determining factor for where we return is largely based on habitual patterns of behavior that have been part and parcel of our lived experience for a long time. For physicians who have developed an identity based almost entirely on "what they can do as doctors" will often do "more medicine" as a means of finding relief. At least their self-image of "who they are" offers strong relief to what they are experiencing in other facets of their lives.

Relief from Quadrant #3

What can you, as a practicing physician knee deep in quadrant #3 activity, do to find genuine relief from the panic and distress that change seems to be causing in your life? Here are some suggestions.

You are exactly where you need to be right now.
Accept this fact as a clear starting point that will enable you to cross the internal bridge to connect with quadrant #1: You are exactly where you need to be in your life right now. This does not mean you want to stay in that place. It means that you are finished with the process of denial and that are open to the lessons that your life is offering you now. Running away and finding relief in all kinds of activity, healthy or otherwise, will not replace nor cannot replace choosing a reflective stance in doing your soul work.

Carpe diem.
Stop beating yourself up with shame, remorse or guilt for what you might label as "lost opportunities." If you never chose them as opportunities nor were open to them as such, all that happened in the past was never an opportunity anyway. This is not as crazy as it might sound. Think of this: only when you are open to listening to the experiences of your life as lessons to be learned is there real opportunity for growth and meaning. Carpe diem. Now that you are open to new life, all that you call the experiences of your past life can be seized, looked at and worked through. Oftentimes you are not able to do it alone, so you may look for assistance from others. Whatever the case, a re-grounding in quadrant #1 will still offer meaning and purpose for even past experiences.

What in you needs to change?
Remove any vestiges from your thinking that change is your enemy. There comes a time when you are called to move away from "not choosing to change" (oftentimes an unconscious event) to "choosing to change" and viewing change as an ally. This does not mean that you change just for the sake of change, not at all. What it means is asking this question and holding your life still enough and long enough to lis-

ten for a response: What in me needs to change so that I might respond creatively and thoughtfully to the situations that my life is presenting to me? Over time you will experience yourself, personally and professionally, re-rooted deeply in quadrant #2 activity. This occurred with a family practitioner named Jack who wanted me to use this story because he felt that there are physicians out there who might benefit from it.

Jack: ...I just don't know how long I can keep up the long hours, the hospital rounds, the many meetings I am required to attend and especially missing out on so much of my family life. My wife is always angry with me, my kids... I swear they don't even know what daddy looks like anymore! Quite frankly, I am beginning to hate what I am doing. I never thought I'd ever think that, much less say it out loud to someone else.

Bill: Is there something specific in your life that you would like to change to make it better?

Jack: (with tears beginning to form) I started to self-prescribe drugs about a year ago just to keep up the pace I was used to when I was younger. I feel guilty as hell – like I betrayed everything I once stood for. Uppers in the morning and throughout the day... downers at night so I could sleep through the pain and deception. Shit, I need help!

Jack is getting help precisely because he got himself out of a denial mode. I spoke with him on the telephone several months after our initial encounter. "I am beginning to reclaim my life," he shared, "and to discover the importance of balance and dealing with change. Today I definitely see with the most clarity I've ever had that meaning and purpose is connected to soul activity and reflected in how I do whatever I do in the world." (Jack, thank you and I do keep my promises.)

A world of alienation and self-destructive behavior (Quadrant #4)

Movement from the generative to the degenerative side of the curve is progressive. There is no leapfrogging from one quadrant to another. Quadrant #4 activity can be summed up in two words: total alienation from quadrant #1 activity. Typically, people who are stuck in quadrant #3 for a long period of time may become vulnerable for an even more progressive deterioration in their personal lives. When destructive, addictive behavior patterns are established in quadrant #4 activity, professional help is most surely needed. The chief characteristics of this quadrant are: total alienation from the life of the soul, a deep-seeded hopelessness, intense feelings of powerlessness and possibly desires for self-destruction. People rooted in quadrant #4, grow into bitter old men and women whose lives have grown so dysfunctional that it would take a Mac truck running them over to get their attention. Even then I wonder if they would be open to change by themselves. Probably not. One of the more effective ways in helping quadrant #4 persons is through a direct intervention, much like the intervention process that is so effective in Alcoholics Anonymous. The intervention has to be direct, forceful, and done by people who care deeply about the person who is suffering. Oftentimes, persons who themselves have been in quadrant #4 at one time make the best interveners.

About change and chaos

In the health care world today, and particular from the perspective of the clinical practitioner, the experience of physicians' ability to change in the midst of seeming chaos contains the capacity for tremendous spiritual growth and creative development. Chaotic conditions can become the bedrock for rediscovering our souls and re-energizing our spirits in ways medical schools, politicians, administrators and the like never dreamed possible. In the health care arena today, we see changes occurring on grand scales almost daily: technologies are evolving, genetic science is discovering new pathways into human evolution, pharmacology seems to be forever on the cutting edge of finding new ways of extending quality of life and eradicating diseases, and the entire system of how health care is delivered and paid for is radically changing. In this cultural and political environment of change and chaos, creativity and spirituality are fast becoming the keys for unlocking the energy needed to deal with the breakdowns in personal and organizational predictability that have characterized the practice of medicine for decades and longer. The tension points that physicians are experiencing are being brought more and more into the light of day, especially in regards to an autonomous, independent practice of medicine. Physician autonomy is becoming an endangered species. Utilization review personnel at the insurance end of health care are literally telling physicians when, how and where to practice their craft. Ownership of physician practices by large health systems and insurance companies, the "de-valuing" of multi-specialty practitioners in favor of primary care practitioners and the way physicians are allowed to refer patients are but a few of the changes evolving today. For some these are threats; for others, opportunities.

Through it all, however, you and I have choices. We can learn ways of taking care of ourselves or not; we can change behavior and attitudes or not; we can discover a new and exciting way to be in health care today or not. The choice is ours to make or not to make. Listen for a moment to Cheryl, a practicing 39-year-old pediatrician from a rural area in the Midwest:

I was not prepared to practice medicine with human beings when I started my residency program. I was trained to learn about life and healing through the study of dead matter, carcasses and corpses. I graduated at the top of my medical school class and had several choices about where I was going to do residency. I remember the first year and being fearful about whether or not I measured up to the standards of the different docs I from whom I was learning with each rotation. That anxiety eventually turned into a bleeding ulcer. After a while things began to even out for me as I got into the routine of long hours with a growing comfort level that I wouldn't kill anyone during my surgery rotation. Towards the end of my pediatric residency, I began to realize how far I had come in honing my diagnostic skills, in developing a strong reliable knowledge base in my specialty. I also began to realize the price I had to pay – how out of control my life was getting. I had no really close friends. All my energies were put into medicine. I was becoming a workaholic. I used to rationalize this imbalance as "the price I had to pay" to be excellent. That defense faded away quickly enough. I continued to struggle emotionally with the effects of distress and the lack of self-care on any level. About a year ago, a nurse in my office and I had lunch together. I confided in her, relating a tale of unhappiness and distress. She looked me squarely in the eye and said: "It sounds to me like you are finally listening to your soul speak and coming to understand your own spirit. Even though it might hurt – much like breaking in a new pair of shoes – you will soon feel a comfort level. For over 20 years I have seen doctors come and go here. You fit the mold, at least until today." I nearly lost my breath – wanting to defend a system that had prepared me so well to be a skilled pediatrician. How could I deny my past? Well, there and then, I decided that I didn't have to. I just had to admit that I knew little about taking care of my spirit – my own self. I think I'm on the path now to discovering "who I am" beneath the role of physician.

Self-Reflection

What is your life asking of you? What are you asking of your life? What in you needs to change? What is it that you want to create in your lifetime – and upon what will you create it? These are the soul questions that need to be asked and listened to no matter what you do, no matter what your age, no matter what.

Case study

"When a dog runs at you, whistle for him"

A regular reader of my monthly newsletter called recently to talk about the difficulty he was having in dealing with all the changes going on in medicine today – both from a clinical and business perspective. After listening intently to him for 15 minutes, I suddenly was reminded of this Henry David Thoreau quote: "When a dog runs at you (and you are afraid of dogs), whistle for him." What follows is this physician's story.

John is a 46-year-old physician who has a very busy family practice in a highly competitive urban area. Three major health systems dominate the marketplace. John is part of a five-person family medicine clinic that was purchased by one of the health systems. John was the last of his partners to go "kicking and screaming" into this inevitable partnership. Competitive factors were working against these physicians staying independent. An idealist by nature, John felt that he would have to sacrifice a lot in order "to be a good soldier" as he put it. Two years into the new relationship had begun to take their toll on John's energy and sense of purpose for practicing medicine. He told me directly: "I am hanging on to my dreams by the slimmest of threads! I now have more people telling me how to practice medicine, when to admit to the hospital and for what reason, when to discharge, when to do this, when to do that. I have never been to so many corporate meetings in my professional life before. I think I am on some kind of blacklist because I seem to have a lot of meetings with the VP for Physician Relations, from the utilization management department of the hospital, and occasionally from the hospital president. Maybe I am getting paranoid, but I swear some of my colleagues avoid sitting next to me at CME presentations."

Today, John is questioning the very existence of his original dream of practicing medicine. What had sustained him through medical school and residency now seemed very far away. He is feeling sharp levels of distress – so much so that he has contemplated leaving medicine and pursuing other ventures in life.

Are you giving away your power?

Our capacity to change is directly related to our capacity to stay connected to who we are, to our power and energy in the depths of our soul. The startling paradox is this: when we truly accept ourselves as we are and the power inherent within our spirit, we are less likely to surrender our power to others or see the demands of change as threats to our well being. Perhaps the way we give away our power is by allowing ourselves to stay depressed, distressed, and in a blaming mode? As I shared with John, to stand in our own power is to see the challenges that are presented to us daily, not as threats but as opportunities and teachers of growth. How have you, in your practice of medicine, surrendered your power to the demands and new configurations of a changing health care world? John, upon further reflection, admitted to me that he felt that medicine had failed him because it had failed to live up to earlier promises. His challenge, as for all of us, is not to be anchored in some ideal image grounded in the past, but to stay anchored in the energy that dreams provide. This motivational energy is not behavior specific all the time. What we do may change over time to meet the demands of new challenges. Real learning occurs when we can take those challenges deep inside our own soul and allow the power of our original dream to breathe new life into what we are doing.

Your mind colors your reality.

Our mind has the capacity and power to twist reality to conform to our beliefs about the way life should be, not accepting life as it is and as it unfolds. On an HBO comedy special, comedian George Carlin uttered a wonderful example of what I mean: "I am not a complete vegetarian. I eat only animals that have died in their sleep!" Another way of looking at this would be to say that our mind projects meaning into any experience. This projection, coming out of our own belief system, colors our reality. I call this the ultimate in control.

Meaning finds you when you are ready.

The opposite of this, and what I encouraged John to consider, is to allow meaning to surface or unfold as a by-product of self-reflection. So, for example, instead of making judgments and projecting blame onto untold numbers of people, a wise physician would take a moment and ask: "What is this experience trying to teach me?" Meaning find us when we are ready and willing to learn the lessons our life holds out to us. Sometimes our best teachers are our perceived enemies, those people who seem to grind on our nerves. For physicians, sometimes teachers take the form of the whitewater rapids of change in the health care world. The key for John, and for us I believe, is to remain open in our souls for new levels of meaning that can deepen our original dreams about our path in this lifetime. All we need to do is confront the "dogs in our lives that are running at us" head on and they will become marvelous teachers for us.

Your Thoughts Along The Way

*(Take a moment to write down any thoughts
or insights you want to remember.)*

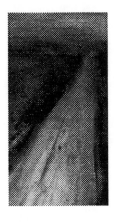

Chapter SIX

MOVING AWAY FROM INSANITY!

I was attending a clinical conference early in 1995, two months before I began writing this manuscript. The theme for the luncheon meeting centered on issues involved in malpractice allegations and the role of the hospital peer review committee. I must have been tired, because I do not remember much from the presenters that day. What I do remember was a beautiful comment shared by a physician who had just gone through malpractice litigation. After telling a little of his story, he got to the punch line: "Experience is not what happens to me; but rather, it is what I make out of what happens to me." That was insightful to me. A true experience cannot be taken for granted. It needs consciousness and some level of meaning. The way this physician learned from his experience in malpractice litigation, a potentially disastrous situation, helped me view the power of choice differently. I began to reflect on how meaning is discovered in life whenever we hold our life still enough and allow the experience to teach us. When we are able to do this consistently, we find that each and every situation life presents us is a teachable moment – and that no situation can overwhelm us unless we allow it to.

We have a personal history filled with a myriad of experiences that have shaped and formed not only our self–image and the way we think, but also our image of the world around us. As part of this personal history, we have formed ideas about reality, work, relationships, and even God. Whether or not we know it consciously, our entire past history has brought us dramatically and powerfully to this very moment in time. This present moment is the only moment available in which to make choices about how our future will unfold, about how the drama of our life will play itself out. This is the real moment given to us to ask basic questions about our life's journey: what is my life asking of me and what am I asking of my life? The way we respond to these questions has the power to reveal a deeper sense of who we are and who we are becoming. These, in a nutshell, are the basic spiritual questions that we all ask, avoid asking, and even when asked, to which we avoid listening. Unpacking these questions has the power to reveal the movements of our life (see chapter 5), that is, the processes and ways we have learned to behave, reason and feel. These moments reveal meaning and purpose no matter what we are doing, whether we enjoy ourselves or not. Meaning is discovered in listening to the question – a by–product of reflection. In fact, I believe these kinds of questions actually drive the spiritual journey toward deeper meaning and purpose.

What is life asking of us? What are we asking of life?

Four thoughts continue to be pivotal for me in reconnecting with my soul power. I think about them whenever I get a gut wrenching feeling my life is moving forward without me, that my life is somehow chugging along without much direction and guidance from within. Pathetically, when I do not ground myself in these four teachings, I end up doing more of what is actually causing the problem in the first place – more work, more avoidance, more rationalizations, less reflective time, etc. I offer these thoughts to you.

You have an inner teacher. Every person born into this world has an inner teacher, an inner guide or leader, that when accessed, can teach the lessons of wisdom, the art of creating a purposeful vision, and can bring a degree of clarity into everyday living.

Stan G. has practiced primary care medicine for over 20 years. Up until two years ago his practice gave him great satisfaction. He characterized himself as a "hard worker who is married to his medical practice." He had lived alone since his divorce six years ago. With no family and few really close friends, practicing medicine was his life. His colleagues, Stan confided to me, saw him as a loner, a label he had also put on himself. About 2 years ago, when Stan was in his mid–50's, he began wrestling with some major issues: whether to affiliate with a large health care network and thereby become an employee, whether to retire thereby rendering the first issue mute, or whether to pursue his dream of being a country doctor. In the midst of these issues, something terrible happened: he was involved in a fatal car accident in which, through his own negligence, a young boy was killed. Unable to deal with the guilt that overwhelmed him, Stan sought the solace of his colleagues. They encouraged him to get back to work as soon as possible ("the pain will pass if you stay busy" kind of advice) and to visit a psychiatrist. Nothing seemed to help Stan. He beat himself over the head harder and more often than his worst enemy ever could. Feeling spiritually bankrupt and emotionally drained, he entertained notions of suicide. Eighteen months after the accident, Stan still had not been able to forgive himself – even though the boy's family had. By this time, his medical practice had dwindled down to almost nothing. Then something remarkable happened. He met a woman in a counseling group in which he was involved, and they hit it off. An occasional lunch led to dates every weekend. After only three months of going together, the woman told Stan she was dying of liver cancer. Stan's comment was, "But you have so much to live for." Knowing Stan's story, the woman turned the phrase back on him, "But you, too, have so much to live for. Find it inside of you to forgive yourself. You have a lifetime ahead of you. So do I, but much shorter than you. Look inside for what you need." Stan began to do just that. He cancelled his appointment with the psychiatrist and went for a long walk. Stan shared an insight he received while walking: "Asking why the accident happened got me nowhere. I realized that the best way I could make amends to this young boy would be to challenge myself to make something out of my life. Perhaps I could make sense out of what happened by recommitting myself to a life of service to others, both within and without the practice of medicine? I needed to respond to that accident. The best way I knew how was with my very life." Through the gentle prodding of his woman friend, Stan eventually traveled over the imaginary bridge from his ego to his soul. He engaged in the real battle for self–forgiveness. For many months, the mind that served Stan so well in his medical practice, turned against him. His ego pursued self–pity, lack of self–forgiveness and feelings of worthlessness. Replaying of the inner tapes from the accident and rehashing his emotional reaction kept Stan from accepting the fact that his deepest self – his soul – had already forgiven him. Once someone (or something) pointed him in the right direction, Stan discovered the wisdom, the love and self–forgiveness that was there all along. Stan came to realize he needed to give himself time to heal. He chose to do a sabbatical and focus on accessing the power and energy of his soul. Stan spent three months at an out–of–the–way cottage by a lake, reading, writing and reflecting. He went back into his medical practice knowing consciously that he could not turn back the clock – but he sure as hell could create a meaningful future for himself, a future that would encompass medical service to countless people in need.

By accessing our inner teacher, the processes and movements of our life can be raised to a more conscious level and thus serve us rather than denigrate us. The values that drive us, the dreams and purpose that guide us, can contain new possibilities for growth and choice. No matter what we do, no matter what is done to us, the energy and power of our soul is available when we are ready and willing to access it.

Your attention empowers your future. Whatever I pay attention to is what I will empower and create for myself, for in my imagination lies a preview of life's coming attractions. To use an analogy: our imagination is like a radio that receives a variety of stations. The station to which we ultimately choose to listen depends upon our choices. We are spiritually attuned when we learn to focus and pay attention to the images that truly serve to nurture life in its many and varied facets. Spiritually–attuned physicians have learned to cultivate images that serve more than traditional medicine. As one physician told me, "It is just as important to do a correct diagnosis of a physiological problem as it is to respect the patient who has it." This physician went on to add, "My personal self–image as a doctor includes treating and listening to the whole person. I am there to serve, not to be served."

What is it that you truly pay attention to in your life's journey? What dreams, motivations, visions drive you each and every day?

What provides you with conscious daily sustenance for what you do in medicine? Do you have a spiritual practice that affirms the cultivation of soulfulness for your journey in this lifetime? What is your primary motivation in the practice of medicine? Is it more than something you do to earn a living – or is it a calling deeply connected to who you are as a person?

Your fear is your teacher. Spiritually–attuned persons have learned that conflicts, fears and problems are truly opportunities for growth and positive change. They have developed the capacity to reframe their experiences as birthplaces for creative insight. For my physician friend Stan, this confronting his experience – no matter how horrible – and facing his feelings of shame, self–loathing and guilt head on; not running from them. In time, Stan learned a profound truth about himself: In stillness, whether alone or with a trusted friend, he could look into the many faces of his fears. He could welcome them as he would a skilled and caring teacher who wanted nothing less for him than growth in wisdom and love.

God is with you. Centuries ago, a gifted theologian and spiritual writer, Meister Eckhart, wrote: The essence of God is birthing. In our rebirthing process, that is spiritual journey, we discover all blessing and meaning. For all eternity, God lies on a maternity bed giving birth. We are all unfinished words in the mouth of God! In using this metaphor of "birthing", Eckhart was inviting people into a much more personal, active, and powerful sense of God. Rather than a transcendent being disconnected with human experience, Eckhart spoke of a God who is imminent; involved in, around and through the whole range of human experience. We tap into this powerful energy when we allow God to accompany us on our spiritual journeys, into the nooks and crannies of our human experience. Allow me to share a story related to this "birthing" God and a fellow named Jack.

Many years ago, an elderly man I had come to know quite well during a summer of community social work in Houma, Louisiana, shared a powerful, influential thought. His name was Jack. He was one of the neighborhood leaders in the section of Houma that St. Lucy's Community Center served. I met Jack the first morning I stepped out of the house I was staying in for the summer. He had lived across the street from the Center for nearly 40 years. Everyone knew Jack. During that span of time, this man – 84 years young and crippled with a debilitating form of arthritis – sat on his front porch and simply smiled and waved to everyone who passed by. I discovered later that people used to go out of their way to wave back at Jack! Being an early riser, I frequently went across the street to share a cup of coffee with this magical and energetic man. He would tell me stories of what it was like to grow up in the South as a black man, of what it felt like to be on the receiving end of so much hatred and prejudice. Jack shared with me his personal history, his spiritual journey, full of richness of spirit, integrity and meaning. I came to realize that this man, with his clear, warm eyes, gentle smile, and striking presence, was someone special in my life's journey.

One morning, about halfway through the summer, I woke up to discover that someone had broken into the gymnasium at St. Lucy's. I stomped over to survey the damage and found an utter mess – paint spilled on the wooden gym floor, chairs smashed to bits, and windows and doors spray painted with graffiti. I went totally berserk! Four letter words spewed from my mouth like lava from an angry volcano. That's when Jack spotted me. He motioned with his crippled arm to come over and said, "Get your ass over here, Bill, and cool off! I can see smoke coming out of your eyeballs." After listening to me complain and blame everyone from God to the actual vandals, Jack took my hand and told me to look him square in the eye. "I have something more important than broken chairs and spilled paint to tell you," he said quietly. To this day, I am most grateful for what that marvelous man shared with me. He said:

"Bill, never forget, that at times like this you must go deep inside of yourself and be willing to see yourself and your life experiences as God sees them. You are exactly where you need to be at this very moment. You cannot always control events, but you can respond to them from your soul – which is yours. Your soul is your power and gift to the world around you, including the vandals. See things the way God sees them and you will soon learn forgiveness, compassion, and the lessons that love has to teach. Whether you and I realize it or not, our heritage and gift of life is dependent on our capacity to respond from our souls to the situations life presents

us. It is not what you can do materially or physically that will afford meaning for you. Long after the gym is cleaned up and the vandals caught, anger will fester in your heart unless you learn what you are supposed to learn. I am not an educated person – no formal schooling for me. But I do know what I know and what works for me. What in you right now, Bill, needs to change to make this situation work for you and not against you? Until you answer that question in your soul, you will never see the opportunity that was given to you for your growth."

I clearly remember leaving Jack that morning, not quite sure of what I had just learned. Something had begun to stir inside of me that would not let go. I went back to my room at St. Lucy's and took out a notebook and began to write. I knew that Jack was meant to share what he had learned in his life with me in order to impact my life. Funny thing – I remember writing about how grateful I was to the vandals for what they had done! Is that crazy or what? The summer of 1970 was the beginning of raising my spiritual journey to a conscious level. To this day, I can still see Jack in my mind's eye, with his wonderful aura and presence, sharing his life's journey with me over the course of that summer.

"I wonder – is God able to find me?"

Several years ago, a Jewish physician sitting next to me in a panel presentation on health care advance directives leaned over and whispered in my ear: "Do you know something that I've been thinking about? I was born into a religious tradition that teaches that life is all about allowing God to find me wherever I am. The key is for me to recognize that reality." I still wonder why he felt he needed to share that thought with me. Maybe I looked harried and stressed out – I do not know. I do know that the thought of "God finding me" stuck with me and would not leave. Several days later, I was spending some quiet time preparing for a talk I was asked to give. My mind turned to what the Jewish physician had shared with me. A question surfaced: "I wonder if God is able to find me amidst all my busyness?" Suddenly, it came to me that my religious tradition, Catholicism, had taught me from little on up that life is searching for God. What a stark contrast –

God searching for me on one end of the spectrum and me searching for God on the other. What would it look like for me to approach my relationship with God from a different perspective than I was used to? Would I recognize that God? Then I met Carl....

Case study

Carl J. is an active pulmonologist in charge of the critical care and ventilator unit of a large, tertiary–care hospital. He and his clinic partners also have a busy respiratory care practice. Carl is driven to succeed at whatever he does and whatever he does, he does with the intention of being perfect. Paying attention to detail has made Carl a proficient doctor. He disclosed to me that if he were to describe his practice behavior and attitude it would be "clinically dispassionate in order to stay focused on the tasks at hand. "A colleague of Carl's once remarked that his CCU and ventilator patients seemed to be treated like abstractions, as clinical challenges for him to pull through. Early on in Carl's practice, several patients died. He took it personally, even though his mind told him there was little or no possibility of their recovery. Having done everything he knew possible for these patients, Carl began to set up an internal wall so that he would not have to feel the sting of his patients' dying. Death became the enemy. Carl's "god" became the findings of medical science and the discoveries of new technologies. He trusted them. Just before I began facilitating an ethics conference, Carl came up to me asked this question: "Are you going to talk about God and those Catholic moral principals the Church is so famous for? If so, I'm out of here."

Self–reflection

Are you open to God finding you?

Perhaps God meets you at the tension points of your life – the death of a patient, the illness of a spouse – or at any of the profound, defining moments of your life. The issue is: are you receptive to God finding you in the midst of these events? Can you recognize, at the very core of who you are, that God may be speaking to you through the events of your clinical practice? Imagine these words from the poet Mary Oliver in her beautiful poem entitled *Waking* in the context of a distressful moment in your life: "Get up, I depend on you utterly. Everything you need you had the moment before you were born." Take it one step further and imagine a loving God echoing these words in the recesses of your soul.

Are you open to your inner teacher?

There is an old saying that my grandmother passed down to me – and was perhaps passed from her grandmother to her: "Bill, you can be certain that when you are severely tested, you have met the teacher." What definable moments are currently testing you as a physician? Can you hold your life still enough to listen and learn from your inner teacher – even when the teacher is severe and exacting? Could your most tension–filled life experiences actually be leading you back to the original source of your life? Are you open enough to recognize and accept the spiritual dimension of your experiences as a physician? In this context, then, the issue is not either medicine or spirituality – but both ... and.

Are you consciously connected?

Life itself is the quintessential escort and preceptor – perfect in every way. When I meet physicians who are conscious of their call to live a meaningful life in the world of medicine, I usually discover people who are living a soulful life, maintaining the oftentimes difficult balance between the demands of the outer world of practicing medicine and the inner world of meaning through self–reflection. How does the busy work in your life impact your staying consciously connected to the source of your power and energy inside? What are you doing to cultivate your spiritual life amid the demands and tensions of your outer world? What would you say to Carl if he asked you for help in dealing with the tensions in his life? In your practice of medicine, do you make time to connect with yourself, and go out into the clinic, office, or hospital with the sacred intention of assisting others? By being still, we remember who we are, and in so doing, God finds us.

Your Thoughts Along The Way

*(Take a moment to write down any thoughts
or insights you want to remember.)*

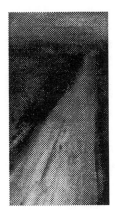

Chapter Seven

"I AM TRYING TO CULTIVATE A LIFESTYLE THAT DOES NOT REQUIRE MY PRESENCE"

I must confess that I am not an avid comic strip reader. Doonesbury is becoming an exception to the rule. Garry Trudeau's biting humor and satire offer me more than just a chuckle and an occasional smile. I am using a quote of his regarding presence as the title of this chapter because too often I have witnessed an absence of presence in health care delivery and leadership. I have seen marvelously intelligent and technologically proficient medical practitioners leave their humanity at the door of the hospital room or in their car in the clinic parking lot. Many of us have been examined by physicians who have treated us more like a diagnostic challenge than a fellow human being. I have witnessed more passion at clinical conferences where physicians have debated treatment options and received a free lunch than I had at my bedside when I was recuperating from hernia surgery.

Why have nurses been the traditional bearers of human compassion and presence at the bedside, while physicians have been the traditional bearers of diagnostic and technological skill? Why, from what I have traditionally witnessed, are many physicians more concerned about curing a disease than caring for an individual? Cannot both take place – or does one exclude the other because of time constraints? How did this apparent "way of doing medicine" actually become a part of many physicians' practice patterns? Too many patients? Demands of the workplace? Do insurance companies and/or health systems require assembly–line medicine as a means of being more proficient? As one physician privately shared with me: "To survive, at some point early on in my practice, I unconsciously began to abstract the person from the disease I was called upon to treat." Could this be the reason why? Maybe?

This same physician affirmed a belief of mine that has been simmering on the back burners of my mind for some time now: years upon years of formal training, from medical school through residency, have been devoted to teaching physicians to cure disease and to alleviate suffering; and only a fraction of time, energy, or formal training have gone into teaching physicians how to care for the people who are diseased or who suffer. In a health care system driven by a paradigm of curing, death quite literally becomes the enemy and tends to create a sense of failure for the physician grounded only in this curing model of health care delivery. For all of us, and especially for physicians who possess skills and diagnostic abilities that relieve suffering, free us from illness, and cure our disease, caring demands a high degree of human presence. In the delivery of good medicine, caring validates and acknowledges the humanness of patients in the context of applied medicine by physicians.

An oncologist, who works daily in a hospice environment, once remarked how some of her patients died rather quickly, once diagnosed with a terminal illness. But others, with even more severe diseases and less prognosticated time to live, stayed alive to finish their assignment on this earth. In so doing, these people had a wonderful, almost heroic, attitude about living and dying. Instead of living in despair and hopelessness, with resignation to their fate, these patients had a most beautiful sense of hope going for them that belied their disease–ravaged bodies. "You would think," she remarked to a group of residents making rounds with her, "that these people had just won the lottery!"

Her homespun belief, based on her clinical experience, concluded: physicians have a wealth of scientific knowledge of applied medicine and have the ability to treat the body's ills, but only the patient possesses the power and energy to work from the inside in the healing process. When both patient and physician are present together, healing works – even if curing is not possible.

How, then, can presence be best described and portrayed in a clinical setting? I have witnessed physicians that are consciously and consistently connected to the source of their own power and energy, their souls. This connectedness enables them to integrate their own humanness, vulnerability, and at times brokenness, with their wondrous medical skills. They bring all of these gifts to the physician–patient encounter. They identify with patients in their humanness and deepening recognition of being partners in a healing process. These physicians believe that there is a spiritual dimension to doing good medicine. Presence is simply soul power to soul power. Presence for physicians is the recognition that physical illness and disease often have a spiritual dimension to them. The oncologist knew that she was a practitioner of spiritual and physiological medicine. One day after leaving her office, she added quietly to me: "Genuine health, not just for hospice patients, but for all patients, is found in the recovery of the soul – from the perspective of both physicians and patients. Words don't do it, but listening and being present does."

When considering the experience of being present to patients, three issues tend to come to mind, especially to those who work in clinical settings. However, I have heard physicians share the following issues in a variety of settings. Each of the comments is connected to the spiritual gift of presence – each offering a different perspective on integrating the value of presence into clinical practice.

"I'm too busy already! All I need is one more thing added to my work load. I barely have time to see my family." (Issue: Time – friend or foe?)

"Are you nuts or something? Why do I need to pay attention to some esoteric book about spirituality? Leave that to the priests and nuns." (Issue: I give power to that which I pay attention.)

"People come to me to be cured. I have the required skills and knowledge. That's what they expect and that's what I get paid for. What else do you want from me?" (Issue: By paying attention to processes in addition to outcomes, we will discover meaning in the context of relationships.)

Time: Friend or foe?

In my personal experience, friends are relationally powerful people. Friends have the capacity to sustain a personal, connected relationship with me no matter what. The relationship is based on both giving and receiving, affecting and being affected. No matter the demands or pressures that exist, friendship is a two–way street that transcends momentary moods, feelings, and time constraints. Foes are people who consciously or unconsciously use me to achieve their own ends and desires. This is little recognition of friendship as a two–way street. It is one dimensional, based on a lack of recognition of who I am. Intuitively, we come to know foes and friends quite easily. With a friend, our lives are enriched, even in small ways. We feel better for having been with them or having shared something honestly with them. Foes, on the other hand, tend to drain our energy. We leave encounters with foes feeling like the air has just been sucked out of our lungs.

We can view time, like a person, as a true friend or a foe. Our experience of time is connected to an attitude grounded in how we view or experience the present moment. For example, we can view time as a foe when trying to accomplish tasks, (so much to do, so little time!), or as a friend when perceived as the opportunity for new life and learning to happen. Time can be our friend in discovering deeper meaning and purpose, in exploring the interior purposes of our souls. From this perspective, time is not necessarily the interval between two points on a linear plane that can be measured; but rather, an experience of the "now" that is being offered. It is precisely the "nowness" of time that presents the gifted moment. Time is a gift that gives an opportunity for presence. In the present moment, there is no past or future, only a timeless sense of now. Time as friend creates the experience of inner groundedness, providing a present that is seemingly beyond limit, where we have new possibilities and choices that can profoundly influence the direction of our lives. The potential of the "now" includes the capacity to change old ways of thinking, to move from old habitual behaviors toward deep thought and conviction, and the ability to respond differently to the belief systems that have been part and parcel of our lives up to this point. The now is ours to grasp, if we choose.

If we apply this relational sense of time to the patient/physician relationship, time becomes a friend, providing the opportunity for a soulful connection and real presence between the physician and patient. It does not take any more "time" for this to occur. What changes is the internal disposition that the physician brings to the encounter. Recently, I went on rounds with a family practice physician. Before he went in the room to visit a patient, he would take the chart out of the wall holder, cross his arms after reviewing it, and take a few deep breaths. I noticed that after seeing the patient, he would put the chart back where it belonged and once again fold his arms and take a few deep breaths. After the third time, I asked him what this moment of quiet was all about for him. Looking me straight in the eye, he said: "Bill, I want to be as present to each of my patients as I am capable of being. After years of treating patients like numbers in a supermarket line waiting to get a cut of meat, I had a patient whose symptoms I missed altogether. She complained of severe headaches. I was in a hurry, so I ordered a neurological consult. The tests came back negative. I saw her six months later and again she was complaining of severe headaches. This time I spent more time with her and discovered that her migraine headaches were connected to allergic reactions to environmental factors. She asked me why she had to suffer for six months when, if I had taken more time with her case, the problem could have been solved back then. That's when I knew I had to change the way I was practicing medicine. The assembly line method doesn't work for this guy anymore!"

I will never forget the conviction with which this physician carried the value of presence. He carried it next to his heart. Each patient encounter became an opportunity for a soulful connection. It was not the disease that this family practitioner was reflecting on, it was the person behind the disease. He let me know that his patients are indeed teaching him to be a healer. Time as friend always has a reflective element to it.

Time as foe can seem like a series of bounded and limited moments, sandwiched in between the past and future, with little or no conscious connection to the meaning that connects all the "now" moments of my life. From this perspective, time is experienced as a series of unilateral moments with little or no reflective, connected sense involved. Time is simply a chance to do, to give, to manipulate. There is a tangible absence of any sense of relatedness that by defini- tion would include both giving and receiving, influencing and being influenced. Time in a relational sense allows us the opportunity to consciously learn from the experiences that life presents. We can reflect on them and discover a sense of meaning and purpose. Time as foe sends energy out into the external world of activity; time as friend sees expended energy returning in terms of being more present to events in the external world of activity. Time as unilateral leads to burn out; time as relational leads to a growing connection of what we do to a larger world of meaning and purpose. The paradox of living relational- ly is that the more we give, the more we get back in terms of meaning and purpose.

The late Dr. Harold Borkawf, a very popular obstetrician and gyne- cologist, was a rare bird indeed. His waiting room seemed like Grand Central Station on Friday afternoon. Every time Peg and I would go to visit him during our pregnancy, I marveled at how he kept his sanity. Not only did Harold have a busy OB/GYN practice, but he served as mentor to more physicians than I probably will know in a lifetime. He had time for people, a relational sense of time that was connected to his vocation of being a physician. While his practice was very busy and demanding, it never seemed hectic. Once he told me that sixteen hour days were the norm sometimes, not the exception. I never felt, in my personal experience with Harold and in listening to stories about him after his death, that time was an enemy for him. I remember a pro- foundly moving question he shared with me: "I have enough to live on even if I stopped working today. I only need a few pairs of pants, shirts, coats and the like. I can only wear them one at a time anyway. Once a person accumulates material wealth and well being, then what"? It was the "then what" that struck me. Harold was referring to his own search for meaning and fulfillment in life. Later, he realized hi "then what" was to return to his native South Africa and work as a pri- mary care physician in the black townships. Whatever he did, I truly believe, was connected to that dream. One day he would return. Until then, everything he did was connected to that purpose. My experience of Harold was truly a gift of great importance. He brought my twin boy and girl, Sammy and Jessie, safely into this world, and he was a profoundly gracious man. As I sit here now, I can imagine him speaking:

Bill, I have always felt appreciative of the time I have to live out my life. I now know how important and precious the present moment is. To discover fundamental meaning and purpose is to realize that the very process of life itself generates joy. I have found meaning not in outward actions or possessions in and of themselves, but in the inner radiant currents of my own being – my soul – and in the relationship and release of those currents into the world, to family and friends, to humanity at large, and ultimately to God. This is the question I see with even greater clarity now: how do I use time and the eternal now in the context of my relationships with family, friends, patients and peers? How I responded to that question was my challenge in life. Now is the only moment I have to be present.

My learning with Harold continues.

I give power to that which I pay attention

Presence is such a powerful concept, experience, and way of living, that I find it difficult sometimes to make it real in my mind's eye. I do know that to experience presence is to know it is there. I believe that overusing words in a variety of contexts waters down their meaning. So, I asked myself for another word that could be synonymous to "presence." For me, that word is "power." In fact, power, presence and love all accurately describe the reality of the energy grounded in our souls.

Our minds have the capacity to broadcast powerful energy. They also determine how we experience the world and what we create. They are like giant magnets, drawing in interpretations of the reality we see, feel, touch and taste. Our thoughts and energy go out into the world, affecting others and affecting us on the rebound. In a sense, we hear echoes of what we put out into the world. My grandmother used to say it in this way: "What goes around comes around!" When we find quality time to hold our lives still for a while and reflect, we are giving our minds a chance to filter our experiences and learn from them, to judge and interpret what we have just seen, touched, felt or sensed. Meaning and purpose are by–products of this interpretive, filtering process. Our conscious minds thinks about things. It is those things that we have the opportunity to breathe deeply into our souls. From out of who we are, then, comes the meaning that nurtures our life. Our souls generate meaning; our minds take that meaning and project it outward, in the form of changed behavior, a renewed attitude, and a more enthusiastic expression of life.

All aspects of life take on a different perspective as meaning unfolds for us, calling us to change and be transformed in light of new information and connections we receive from within. The activities that we now perform (our professional functions, for example), are performed more mindfully and carefully because they are seen in the light of an ever–evolving sense of meaning and purpose. A web of meaning is created that connects our present experience to the interior promptings of our soul. Our soul creates a larger world or context for living that energizes us. The larger world or context has meaning and purpose. To be truly present, to be a presence, is to stand in that energy of personal meaning as we each have come to know it for ourselves. That higher purpose influences our thinking and doing in the world. The dreams that guide us become powerful instruments for us each and every day. The magic that happens when we are present allows us to keenly recognize that the people we encounter each day (for example, our patients) are also on a spiritual journey. We can then make the connection that meaning and purpose are not discovered in isolation, but in relationship with others, within community. We also begin to realize that our search for meaning can be enhanced by others but never controlled by them – unless we surrender our power and go off our path onto another's. Each of us is exactly where we need to be in our respective lives. That is our starting point.

Albert Einstein once wrote something wonderful that caused me to think about the power within each of us. He said: "in my imagination contains the preview of my life's coming attractions." If we want a glimpse into our future, all we need is consciousness of the images we carry inside. Our imaginations are powerful gifts, instruments, that sometimes enhance our lives and sometimes detract from them. The thoughts and images in our mind are changing hundreds of times a day perhaps without even being aware. These images are pictures of reality that we hold in our minds. We bring them forward into the present due in large part to our past experiences. We use them as prisms or models with which to judge whether we are good, or how to deal with the situations our life presents. Most importantly, however, these inner images quite literally create our boundaries and limits. How often have we heard ourselves say: "I can't do that", or "I've never done it that way before", or "that's just not me." Take, for example, the images we carry regarding ourselves – our self–images. These self–images are changing fairly constantly depending on the external situations of our life. These self–images are often very subtle and are determined by and large by the inner tapes and scripts that are being replayed from our past. "I'm not worthy to receive such an award," or "how can he/she really love me?", or "this is overwhelming and I can never do it!" come from our self–image voice inside. Why are some people more risk takers than others? Why can some people accept challenges while others shy away? Our particular response to these and similar questions rests with our self–image. The ways we have habitually responded to events, situations, and people in life, conditions us and writes scripts in patterns particular to each of us. Our thoughts and reactions to events, situations and people have been reinforced over and over again through our history. For example, when we are confronted with an authority figure, our inner script pops up on the computer screen of our self–image and conditions our first response. In a fraction of a second, our preconditioning will take over and our internal reaction to the authority figure will be consistent with the reactions we have had with all the authority figures in our past.

These inner tapes or scripts, in large part, go into forming the images of ourselves that we have at any given moment. What is important to note here is that we have the capacity to change these tapes whenever we choose to do our interior work – our soul work. The key ingredient that goes into that change process (changing a particular self image that is not life giving) is awareness – a conscious connection to our thought processes and acceptance that this self image is not working for us. The change process can begin whenever we find ourselves saying things like "I don't like myself very much for the way I reacted to this situation" or "Here is another authority figure. Why do these people seem to single me out for something or other?" Having said this, however, I would say that for the most part our self image moves around on an unconscious level and is difficult to become aware of initially. One way of becoming aware of our self image is to confront ourselves about what we believe our limitations are. Our image of self sets our limit. The way we think about ourselves at any given moment will indicate the way we feel about ourselves. How we feel about ourselves (confident, strong, weak, misunderstood, etc.) will often determine our behavior in external circumstances. Simply put, the images of self we carry around inside of us determine and condition our responses to the demands of life.

Our self images can either serve our life well or detract from it. For example, as physicians, what images of being doctors are being played and replayed in our clinical practice these days? Where did our inner sense of being a doctor come from? Have we ever taken the time to challenge the tapes and scripts that seem to be governing our practice of medicine? These are important questions in our search for meaning in life, in what we do, in how we do it, and how we respond to change. Once we get to a place in our life where we have a desire to change because something or other is not working too well in our life, then we have gotten to the very internal place that requires reflection on the images we carry around inside. As we become aware of those images that serve our life, we put ourselves in a marvelous position to consciously cultivate and nurture those positive, life–serving ones and conversely, to let go of those that do not. Our behavior as physician, writer, father and mother, will flow from those very images.

What images are conjured up when we think of the words "spirituality" or "spiritual journey?" With whom do we associate those words? A rabbi, a priest, a nun, a holy person of some sort? Do we have room in our own book of self images to include ourselves on that list? If not, why not? For some people, the very mention of the word "spirituality" connotes an association with religion or some kind of religious experience. For others, a sense of unworthiness leads them to believe that spirituality is reserved for special people – certainly not for busy physicians. Let me suggest a description of spirituality that includes all of us, no matter what our calling in life is. Spirituality is a process of growing into wholeness, a process of coming to power – a power that is grounded deeply in the soul and connected to a conscious uncovering of meaning and purpose. At the very core of who we are rests a dynamic energy of personal power. The spiritual journey is simply the acknowledgment of that power and the allowing of it to become evident in our life. In other words, we are all born with a spiritual nature, meant to be developed and brought forth. Unlike a religious tradition that we might be born into because of our family of origin or adoption, our spiritual nature does not come to us from the outside. It is part and parcel of who we are at birth – irrespective of a particular religious tradition.

While religion can play a very pivotal role in our lives, it is not the same as spirituality. Our religious symbols, prayer forms, and teachings are meant to serve our spirituality – not the other way around. Religion, I would suggest, can be a way of getting there, not the final destination or end in and of itself. To the extent that our religious faith serves to enhance and enliven our spirituality, it will be relevant. As we pay more and more attention to the spiritual dimension of our life, we will be empowering that energizing center (our soul) to work for us as we live out our everyday life. Our religious faith can be an integral part of connecting to the source of meaning and purpose in our life. The more we befriend and stay connected to that power (Power), the more we can count on its exploding into the far reaches and corners of our life. Even in the darkest hours of our experience, there is a power there that enables us to grow through whatever life is presenting to us. It is this inner dimension of our life that will say to us in times of crisis and even chaos: "You are exactly where you need to be. This moment might be an exacting teacher, but it is your starting point. It is where you are being asked to bring forth the power of your soul that you were born with." We literally give power to that which we pay attention.

Paying attention to outcomes and process helps us to discover meaning in the very context of relationships.

Back in 1983 when I was doing consulting work in the areas of personal growth and organizational development, one of my clients was a very wealthy businessman who really had a hardball knack for making money. He was indeed a person with a Midas touch. As an entrepreneurial businessman, his fortune grew from nothing to a company that employed over 250 people at its peak. Lavish office space, an executive dining room with a chef, and many other trappings of success, were amply evident. To the same degree that this man was successful in making a fortune, he was unsuccessful in relating to people. Meaning and purpose fluctuated with his company's bottom line. This business man (whom I will call Dick) telephoned me one day saying that he had heard I did good work in helping organizations "shape up their personnel and get rid of the dead wood." (Those were his exact words.) I agreed to do consulting work at his company, but not the way he thought I would. During an initial face to face meeting with Dick, I shared with him the conditions under which I would accept this assignment. He would have to adhere to them rigorously or else I would quit in a heartbeat. Following were my conditions:

1. Dick had to agree to undergo and experience some rather drastic lifestyle changes for a period of five consecutive working days. These changes included: a) wearing a sport coat instead of a $600 Italian made three–piece suit; b) riding a bus to and from work, which meant leaving the Rolls Royce in the garage; c) leaving all credit cards at home and carrying no more than $10 cash at any one time; d) bringing his lunch from home and eating it in the employee dining area and not the executive dining room; e) stopping in a local bar after work that was frequented by many of his employees; and finally, f) calling me on the phone every night to talk about his personal experiences that day.

2. The financial arrangement consisted of this: if Dick quit on the first day, he would owe me $5,000 for services rendered; if he quit the process on the second day, he would owe $4,000; if on the third day, $3,000; if on the fourth, $2,000; and if he lasted the whole week faithfully, he would owe me $1,000. I somehow knew this arrangement would get and keep his attention.

3. If Dick had a business luncheon scheduled for that week, he would have to bring enough food from home for the others. No running out to the club and starting a tab.

I still don't know why Dick said "yes" to these conditions. My gut feeling tells me he was intrigued with the challenge. I knew underneath it all that money was not the great generator of meaning that Dick assumed it was. Early on in our initial meeting, I began to sense that Dick was a lonely man who knew the ways of the world, but knew precious little about the path to his own soul. That was, after all, the real reason he accepted this challenge – only he did not know it consciously at that time.

A whole lot of learning went on that week for both of us. I even looked forward to the regular 8:00 p.m. phone calls from Dick. Although he was quite nervous at the start, he gradually warmed up to what I was asking of him. What follows are some of the major lessons we both uncovered that week. What started as a week from hell for Dick, soon evolved into a slow understanding of his spiritual path in life.

> * *There are people, events, and situations in our lives that call us to either emerge from our cocoons or become more rooted in them. The key is whether or not we are open to learning from our experiences.*

"I was damn uncomfortable today, bordering on goddamn embarrassment. I kept thinking to myself that this shit too will pass." So began Dick's conscious spiritual journey. From the very start Dick felt terribly distressed and wondered if this project was too much for him. He looked for excuses to get out. What kept him hanging in there that first day was the thought of the $5,000 that it would cost him for me to do nothing at all for him. "What the hell," he said. "I might as well give it a shot and swallow my ego." First thing Monday morning he asked his wife for a ride to the bus stop. They both looked at each other in bewilderment. "Where in the hell are the bus stops in the suburbs?" After calling the bus company's schedule hot–line, Dick got a ride to the nearest bus stop from his wife. She could not stop laughing as he nervously twitched in the front seat. Upon arrival, he stood there waiting for the bus to come along with four other commuters. "I stood there, feeling really awkward, not knowing what to say. I avoided eye contact like the plague. Just as I was resigning myself to a fate worse than death, someone asked me for change. I gave it to her just as the bus arrived. Little did I know that I had just given away the change I needed for the bus. I didn't realize that bus drivers don't give change. Fortunately, a nice man behind me gave me the money I needed and said I could pay him back tomorrow." In an increasingly softer tone of voice, Dick began to share how beautiful that experience was, reminding him of the Bible story of the Good Samaritan. As the bus crept along towards his office, a few employees boarded. He recognized their faces, not their names. To his utter amazement, they came over and sat across the aisle from him. They introduced themselves. "I think," Dick relayed to me, "that these folks were shocked to see me riding public transportation. I was sure this experience would be fodder for the gossip mills at the office."

As Dick walked from the bus stop to the front of his building, he mustered up the courage to ask his bus–riding employees what they did at the office and what their names were. (Incidentally, by the end of the week, he and his fellow commuters would be working out a car–pooling arrangement.) As Dick entered the executive office suites, his vice–presidents (or "ass kissers" as he privately referred to them) swarmed around him like bees to honey. Later in the week, he would tell them all to wear sport coats around the office and to bring their own lunch, closing the executive dining room as an exclusive place and opening it up for all to use. Several months later, a contest was held and the lunch room was renamed the "Brown Bag Emporium." Anyway, back to Dick's story of the first day....

Every place he went, Dick sensed that people were staring at him, especially in the lunchroom. (I assured Dick that they were staring at him, probably with mouths open in amazement.) Finding a table was a problem because the lunchroom was a tad small for so many eating at the same time. Dick met a lot of new people – at least new to his experience. Carrying on conversations with them that ranged from how well the Green Bay Packers were doing to stories about their personal lives, he soon began to feel like a sponge overloaded with water. Dick actually began to enjoy the experience of expanding his horizons and meeting people. He told me that it reminded him of his own grow-ing up and working weekends at a hardware store. Lunch times were always occasions to swap stories and get to know people.

The rest of the workday was uneventful. Dick, however, started to laugh a bit over the phone as he recounted his initiation at the local bar near the office complex. "I ordered an Absolute vodka martini, straight up and very dry. The bartender had to ask me how to make a martini. The vodka tasted like wood alcohol. No Absolute. I have decided to order a beer tomorrow." He sat and conversed with some people who may or may not have worked for him. By this time, after two wood alcohol martinis, he really did not care where they worked. He was enjoying himself. One of the people at the bar offered him a ride home after learning that they lived fairly close to each other. Two martinis did not allow Dick the luxury of finding a bus stop.

* *Whenever I forgive myself and remember who I really am, I will be present to bless every person I see and in so doing will allow myself to be blessed.*

As the week progressed, Dick stayed the course and his learning began to take root. People, including his wife and children, were not used to seeing him change his lifestyle and daily routine so dramatically. Their reactions caused Dick to do some introspection. He was not used to the feelings of warmth, acceptance, and sheer delight that were surfac-ing inside. The more he witnessed the human side of his employees, the more he experienced his own. The beauty of the process, as he was able to articulate later on, was that no one forced him to do what he was doing. The process was his choice. Dick told me that as the week went on, he felt a naturalness about the changes he was undergoing. They were not fake or contrived. He was aware of stirrings deep inside. One such experience that had a profound influence on him occurred on the fourth day of the grand experiment. During our nightly conversation on day two, I began to suggest to Dick that he might want to work on developing a sense of presence with some of his employees – just intu-itively walking around the office taking in the environment, feeling and thinking about what he sees. If someone or something strikes you, take time to receive it into your heart and hold it there for a moment. If it involves another person, perhaps offer him or her a cup of coffee and see if they would like to talk. I suggested that what they talked about was not as important as Dick's ability to stay open to what the experience was trying to teach him. Nothing significant happened on day three. On day four, however, while making his "intuitive rounds," he noticed one of his executive vice–presidents looking frazzled, tired, and worn out. Sitting on his leather chair, elbows on the desk, and head in his hands, this young man looked catatonic as he stared out of the window. Dick entered his office, shut the door quietly, and sat down at a chair adjacent to the VP's desk. Out of the blue came these words: "I have to resign, sooner rather than later. I have nothing more to lose."

Caught off guard by the forceful and surprising revelation, Dick kept his composure and asked the man if he wanted to talk for awhile. The VP went on to share with Dick some of the stressors he was feeling on the job – deadlines, productivity levels that seemed unrealistic, the 14–hour days. He shared with Dick how his family life was crumbling and the threats his wife was making about divorce unless something changed. It all seemed to be coming to a head with the VP that morning. Dick continued to listen to this man's story. (Keep in mind, listening was never a high priority for this autocratic, unilateral corporate executive.) At some point, Dick began to talk about his own failed marriages (two) and the current one that was shaky at best. He assured the young man that his job was not in jeopardy and that he should take some time off to take care of himself. Several weeks later, sensing a friendship with Dick, this VP confided that he was using cocaine and drinking more than usual to mask the pain. As Dick shared this part of his experience weeks later, I noticed a quiver in his voice and his eyes welling up with tears. "Are you close to tears, Dick," I asked. "Yes. This person is becoming like a mirror for me ... I see so much of me in him, not only when I was his age, but even now. I never used drugs, but I did use my addiction to work to cover up much of the pain I was feeling personally. I figured that if I worked harder, somehow life would get better. Isn't that a crazy thought? I'm beginning to discover that I've squandered so much time and energy in making money, that the very thing I wanted – love and a family – got buried in the heap. One thing I did know about myself: I knew how to build a business and make it succeed – even believing that I could do it with sheer willpower."

* I will need time to forgive myself. If I don't, I will keep running away and the same old patterns will develop – different people, same old patterns.

This learning was a direct quote from Dick, made several months after we started working together. "I feel so ashamed for all the pain and suffering I've put people through because of my own lack of awareness. Maybe one day these same people will be able to forgive me ... I don't know. The greatest gift I have given myself, however, is the capacity and willingness to be present to others – and to myself. Even more so now, I know what is meant by the saying: I am exactly where I need to be. That so–called week from hell was the starting point for change to happen." Dick taught me that the gift of presence can open doors that even a jackhammer is unable to open.

Postscript: In the weeks and months following my initial involvement with Dick and his organization, I met regularly with him and some of his leadership people. On occasion, he would invite me in to do an in–service program of one sort or another. What Dick was doing – and by now he was becoming more aware of it – was attempting to integrate his own spiritual learnings into the work environment. Clearly, he was tired of developing a lifestyle that did not require his presence. While Dick returned to some of the trappings of his lifestyle, he was on a conscious spiritual journey now that did not trap him into thinking he was somebody he was not. To this day, Dick has a healthy, relationally powerful work style and friendships. He and his wife became proud parents of their first child in 1986.

"THE POWER OF PRESENCE: WHAT CANNOT BE TAUGHT IN MEDICAL SCHOOL"

A physician friend of mine, the chief medical officer at a large tertiary care hospital, recently shared this thought with me: "If I notice myself not being present to my patients and treating them as abstractions or a disease classification, I take time to reflect. One of the best times for a busy physician to reflect about the power of being present is when older patients describe their bowel habits!" He was sharing in a humorous way how vital it is for him to examine his practice of medicine in relationship to the power and energy inherent in being truly present – mentally, emotionally, spiritually and physically – to each human encounter. My friend added, "The single most valuable tool that I have as a physician is the power of being truly present to each patient encounter. When I am, all my skills are brought into play. And you know what? I also learn the art of healing."

Case study

M.L., a 41–year–old internist with a busy practice, recently was admitted to the hospital for an appendectomy. He was readmitted a week later due to a severe infection that required a brief hospital stay. M.L. had never been hospitalized before. Twice in one week was enough for him. Nurses pricked his arm for blood, med techs performed all the standard tests that he had so often ordered for his patients, the surgeon spent time going over the same ground of his personal medical history that the nurse had already done that morning, and the anastesiologist merely repeated what the surgeon had asked two hours previously. Through it all, M.L. kept his patience and experienced with relative good humor all the things his own patients experienced when they were in the hospital. After surgery, despite a sore throat from the intubation and soreness due to the Foley tube, his spirits were good. The infection cleared up enough for him to be discharged. Back at his office, M.L. noticed (really for the first time) a plaque on the wall of the waiting room that said, "Respect comes from the Latin word *respicere*, which means the willingness to look again." Taking the plaque down and into his office, M.L. contemplated his recent hospital experience in light of the question, "What can I learn from these experiences?" Later that day, at a consult with a cardiovascular surgeon regarding one of his patients, M.L. said, "I'm learning what it means to be present to my patients, to respect them as individuals, and to allow them to teach me what I need to learn about being a more empathetic physician." The surgeon had no idea what M.L. was talking about.

The power of presence. The power of presence means we have the capacity to engage ourselves intellectually, emotionally, spiritually and physically with the person we are with or the situation in which we find ourselves. The ability of physicians to be present with patients and peers demands the cultivation of soul power – the residence of the power of presence. It means choosing to be present and visible and not drifting off into our own thoughts and assumptions. How often do you experience yourself "not being all there" because you still have not detached from a past problem or emotional conflict? In what experiences in your life as a physician do you seem to "not show up" energetically? When do you find yourself so bored and uninterested that all you can think of is something in the past or what you will be doing ten minutes from now? The power and energy of being present comes from a cultivation and consciousness of soul.

Your soul power is medicine. Native peoples of North and South America historically use the words "power" and "medicine" interchangeably. If we are truly present to someone intellectually, emotionally, spiritually and physically, we are said to be "full of power" and "expressing our medicine." Isn't it curious how the meaning of the word medicine is used – being full of power? Have you, as a practicing physician, ever considered that "your medicine" goes way beyond what you learned in medical school or what you continue to learn through reading, research and consultation? Consider this for a moment: your original medicine, that is, the personal power of your spirit and soul that you bring into your clinical practice, can never be duplicated anywhere on this earth! Do you believe as strongly in your "original medicine" as you do in the technologies, diagnostic skills and scientific breakthroughs that guide you each day as you practice medicine?

When do you give away your power? As you reflect on your current practice of medicine, the patients in your care, and the colleagues you are connected with – when and with whom do you not bring your "original medicine" to bear? Are there certain people and/or situations that spark your lack of courage in bringing forth this original medicine? Where in fact do you lose your power of being present? In what ways do you respect and honor yourself and others? Have you developed an honest awareness of your limits and boundaries as a physician – as well as those of the other people in your life? Perhaps as you are listening to the recounting of your next elderly patient's bowel habits, these questions will surface? As usual, the choice is yours.

Your Thoughts Along The Way

*(Take a moment to write down any thoughts
or insights you want to remember.)*

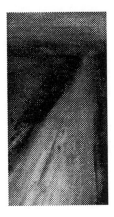

Chapter Eight

THE ROLE OF EMPATHY

"The secret of teaching is not to bring empathy to medical practice, but to keep it there despite the rewards of technology!"

I borrowed this quote from a sentence I read in a marvelous book entitled Empathy and the Practice of Medicine, published under the auspices of the Program for Humanities in Medicine, Yale University School of Medicine. The subtitle of this book, "Beyond Pills and Scalpel," says a lot about the focus of the 17 essays that are contained in it. Looking at what is at the heart of the practice of medicine, the authors speak about the immense value and importance of empathy.

Before we can describe the value of empathy, like most feelings and experiences, we must have first felt and experienced it. To help us do that, I would like to share a wonderful time I had several years ago with second–year medical students studying at the Medical College of Wisconsin. I was asked to assist these young men and women in learning and developing listening skills as they began writing out patient histories for a class. As you read through the description of this event, I encourage you who are caregivers to reflect on your own set of experiences with patients.

All of the students did a fairly good job of recording patient histories. Each afternoon the students and I would gather back in a classroom to share their experiences of the morning. Soon, I began to notice an interesting phenomenon: while the students did a good job in recording what they heard, it did not take long for them to begin referring to their resident in the abstract and in the medical jargon of disease classification. "Sally" in particular exemplified what I mean.

Sally:*/ (taken directly from her script of the interview): "Mrs. Jones in room 416 is an 86–year–old woman who has been at the nursing home for over four years. Her eldest daughter, Marie, admitted her because of a need for extensive rehabilitation due to a total hip replacement. She is suffering from the early stages of Alzheimer's disease so it was difficult obtaining a lot of recent history from her. She is mildly disoriented, complaining of feeling lonely. Mrs. Jones did, however, have a great deal to say about her distant past, growing up on a farm with five brothers and two sisters. She is the sole survivor of this large family. She loves flowers, especially roses and petunias. Her best friend is Amy who is in 418. Mrs. Jones is bedridden and unable to move about the home without the aid of a wheelchair. Outside of the normal aches and pains of old age, 416 is a classic case of a lonely woman who is being farmed out to a nursing home by a family who doesn't visit too often."

Bill: You said, "416 is a classic case." Did Mrs. Jones lose her name since we started?

Sally: Oops! I meant to say Mrs. Jones. I would also add that she basically sits in her room for most of the day staring at the TV. Sometimes Amy joins her. Three times a day she goes to the same dining room as the nursing home tube–feeders.

Bill: (interrupting again) Did you say "tube–feeders?" Have they also lost their names or perhaps they have assumed a new identity?

Sally: I'm sorry. I guess I am taking a few shortcuts ... shouldn't do that I guess.

Bill: I suppose if this were a hospital, we would be talking about the gall bladder in 213, the hearts on the fourth floor, and the crazies on the psych floor!

How easy it is to refer to people by their disease or procedure. As the patient gets abstracted into oblivion, so does the physician's capacity to empathize. Technology and analytical skills meet diagnostic challenges. Empathy and understanding meet caring opportunities for physicians. Empathy demands seeing the whole patient – not just a part of the anatomy.

For our purposes here, I would like to describe empathy as the capacity to project my heart, mind, and soul into the experiences of another person, thereby truly understanding that experience and the person behind it. To better understand both the concept and experience of empathy, I have created a visual aid (see fig. 8:1) that attempts to portray the processes and elements involved in an empathetic relationship. Empathy has the capacity to act as a bridge between the physicians and patients, enhancing relationships as well as diagnostic processes from the perspective of both physicians in diagnosing and patients in telling their presenting symptoms and larger life story.

Fig. 8:1—Empathy as Diagnostic Skill

The Physician/Patient Encounter: What each brings to the table

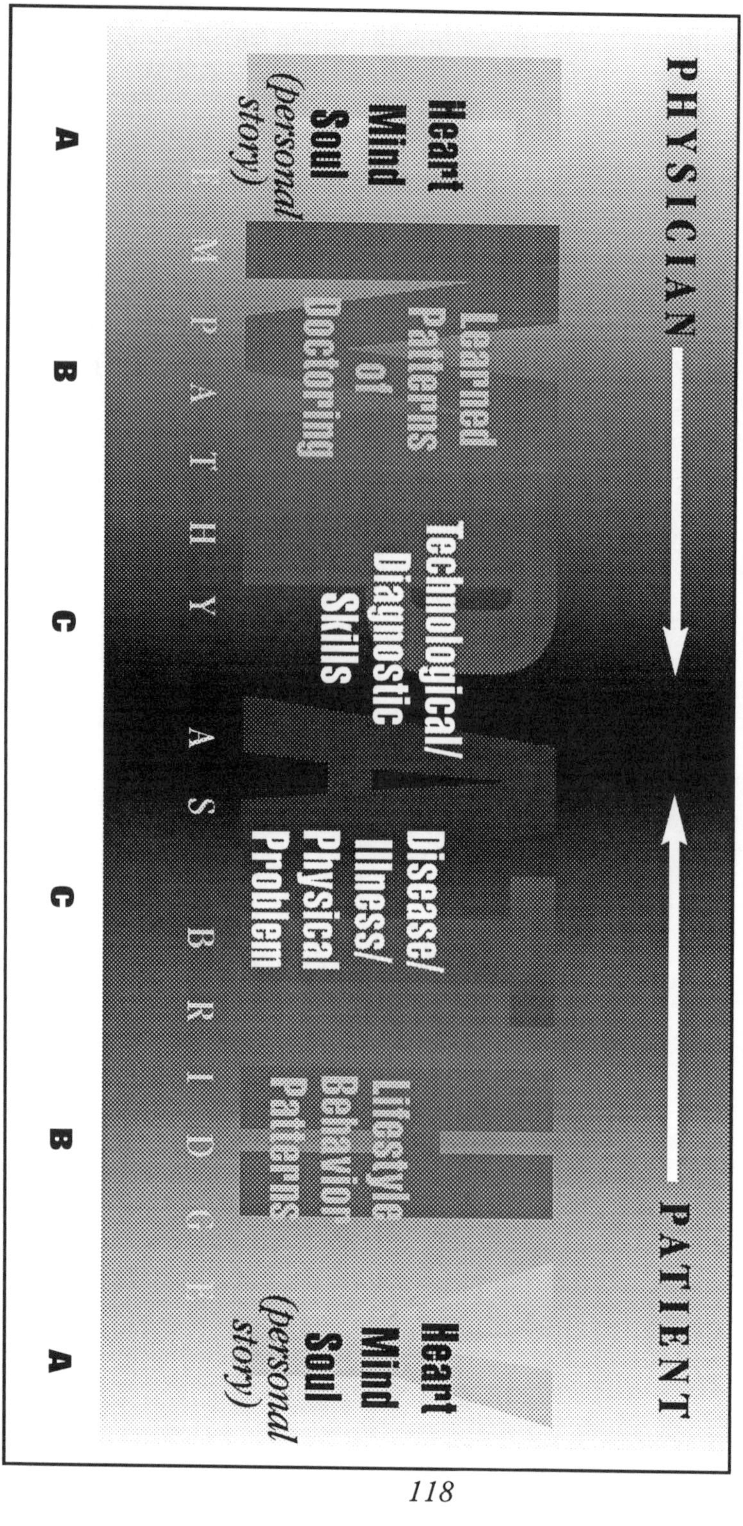

PHYSICIAN

Heart
Mind
Soul
(personal story)

Learned
Patterns
of
Doctoring

Technological/
Diagnostic
Skills

EMPATHY AS BRIDGE

Disease/
Illness/
Physical
Problem

Lifestyle
Behavior
Patterns

Heart
Mind
Soul
(personal story)

PATIENT

A   B   C   C   B   A

Using figure 8:1 as a backdrop, let us use slow motion to describe the process of the empathetic practice of medicine or its lack. Using the examples of new patients, physicians normally are initially confronted with the presenting symptom, disease, or illness – whatever it is that brought the patient to the doctor in the first place. Appropriate questions are routinely asked in an attempt to diagnose. Vital signs are taken; eyes, ears, and throat are examined. All relevant information is noted on the patient's chart. A referral may be made to a specialist; a blood test and/or x–ray may be needed to assist in the proper diagnosis. If a prescription is needed, one is given. A nurse or lab assistant may call later with test results. The physician may also have to place a call to share pertinent information with the patient. Give or take a few steps in the process, any physician who has completed medical training and is qualified can do the above. This is routine. Using the graphic, this encounter describes letter C for both physicians and patients – nothing more, nothing less. From the perspective of empathy, what is missing from this example?

Referring to figure 8:2, we readily can see that the physician and patient are both grounded in their respective Cs in the above case. The dotted line encompassing both Cs represents the extent of a physician/patient encounter that is void of empathy. This invisible boundary line can become the routine definition of the practice of medicine for those physicians who do not consciously attempt to bring empathy into their clinical practice.

Fig. 8:2—Empathy as Diagnostic Skill
The Physician/Patient Encounter: What each brings to the table

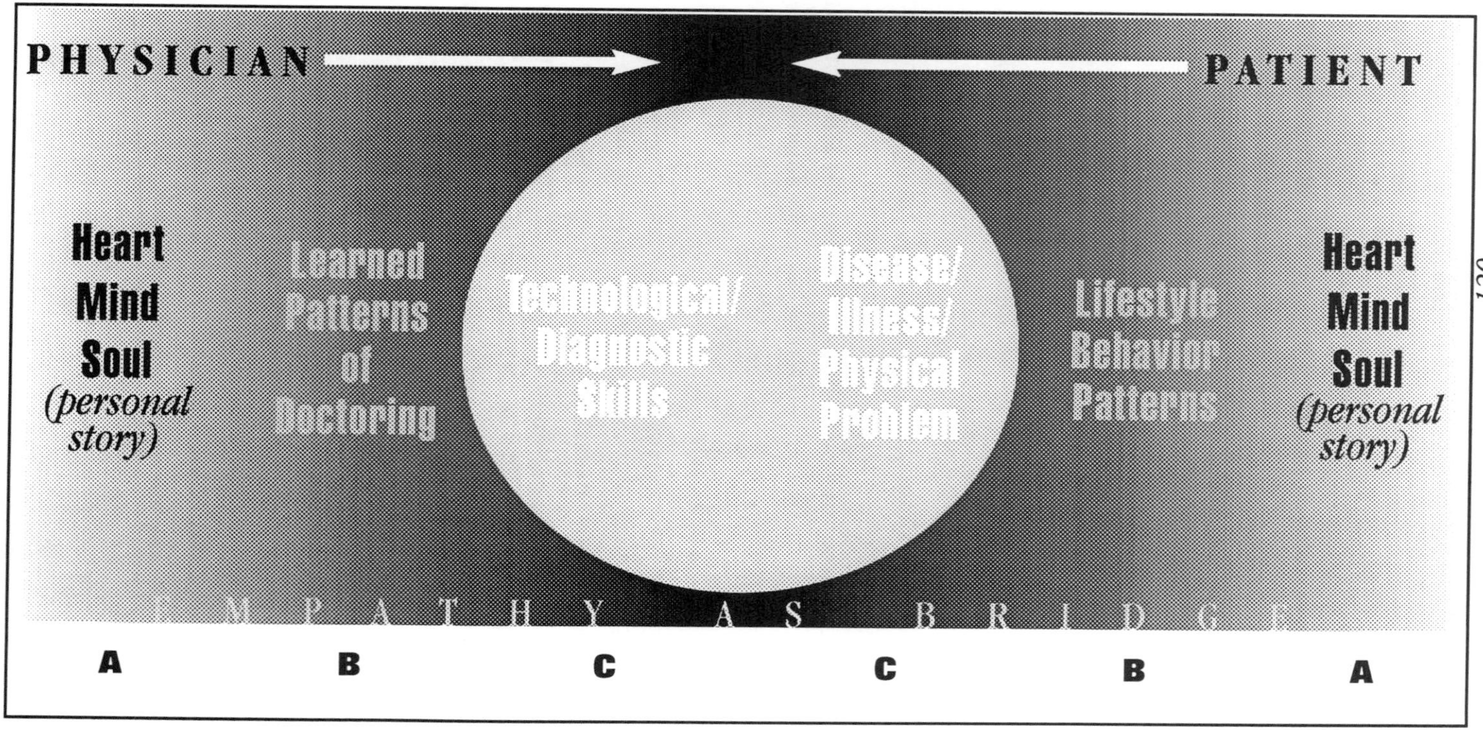

PHYSICIAN

Heart
Mind
Soul
(personal story)

Learned
Patterns
of
Doctoring

Technological/
Diagnostic
Skills

Disorder/
Illness/
Physical
Problem

Lifestyle
Behavior
Patterns

Heart
Mind
Soul
(personal story)

PATIENT

EMPATHY AS BRIDGE

A   B   C   C   B   A

Over time, physicians learn habitual ways of doing doctoring that seem to fit them. They learn the art of doing medicine (category B). These more experienced physicians, grounded in their Bs, have the knack of encouraging their patients to bring out their own Bs – elements of their lifestyle and behavior patterns that might be at the root of their presenting symptoms. For example, physicians who are aware of their own stressors in life (for example, little or no self–care, over-working, or feelings of powerlessness in relationships) and have taken steps to make significant changes in these lifestyle patterns, have a deeper sensitivity to the same dynamics in their patients. These more self–aware physicians are able to integrate into their patient diagnosis a more comprehensive assessment of the non–physical elements that might be contributing to the presenting illness.

Life–Style Behavior Patterns or, "I've always done it this way!"

The pursuit of external power or control can lead to a repression of emotion. To the degree we engage in controlling others (and events), we also disconnect from our own source of power (soul) and hence from the feelings and emotions that make up who we are in any given moment. To assess whether this is true, think of a situation wherein you were trying to win or succeed over someone, for example, an argument you had with someone. We often position ourselves to "get the best of the situation," blocking out any awareness of what the other feels. We feel we are right and, damn it, why doesn't that other person recognize it. If people are close to us, we often block feelings and emotions that are part of our relationship with them. In blocking our feelings, what actually wins are the feelings of anger or frustration that led up to the argument. Whenever we clearly intend to win an argument, we subordinate our feelings about the other in order to control the situation. How often have we experienced ourselves saying something like: "I don't know what got into me. I just lost it. My frustration and anger were disproportionate to the situation." In my experience, when I pursue control over others I will repress my emotions to some degree. If I don't, I appear weak and out of control.

Another powerful, more specific example is the movie *The Doctor*, starring William Hurt. This wonderful story typifies the experience of being held hostage by the medical profession. Hurt's character, a prominent physician, has been diagnosed with cancer. As a rather dispassionate doctor, he now has the tables turned and is the patient. The story evolves around coming into awareness of what it feels like being held hostage – or being controlled by the health care system. The "doctor" is subjected to treatment by his colleagues that he never knew existed. For the first time, as the story unfolds, he becomes personally aware of what it feels like being a patient and being controlled by every level of the medical profession. At the end of the movie, the "doctor" undergoes a marvelous transformation that has profound effects in his own medical practice. The character discovers that the art of being empathetic and practicing medicine with empathy is an integral part of who he is as a physician. Using Fig. 8: 2, A, B, and C are brought into his medical practice.

Whenever empathy is left out of the practice of medicine, a distancing dynamic occurs within physicians. This distancing dynamic eventually closes the door to vital currents originating in physicians' souls that activate and energize their thoughts and actions towards others. The fully human dimension characterizing the physician/patient relationship gives way sooner or later to a more roboticized version of practicing medicine. Physicians in this place lack awareness of their emotional life and cannot associate the effects of anger, sadness, depression, joy, happiness, or grief within their own lives, much less with the lives of their patients. Without personal affirmation of the value and importance of feelings and emotions – and the acceptance of those feelings and emotions as valid participants in the physician–patient encounter – physicians themselves, like all of us, will lose something quite extraordinary in their professional lives. How can we project empathy if we do not know the emotion of empathy within ourselves? If physicians lose the ability to witness their own emotional lives and deny that their emotions are valuable assets in the practice of medicine, then what becomes of the human dimension of medicine? What will become of healing when treating patients is not enough? What will happen ultimately to the souls of physicians when they leave empathy out of their practice of medicine? What will happen to the patients through all of this?

For physicians, empathy can become the bridge that leads away from using patients to feed self–esteem, ego, or economic needs toward an abiding sense of being present to and understanding patients from the inside out, that is, seeing them as persons with a personal history. Empathy is a heart, mind and soul connection with the essence of each patient encountered. It can become a personal contract between the physician and the patient that honors the physiology and interior life of both. Empathy pays great attention to the process of doing medicine, that is, to how physicians diagnose patients' maladies, to the way in which a surgeon speaks with a patient before and after surgery, to the way a gynecologist touches a patient during a pelvic exam. Empathy has an inherent healing power attached to it as it is expressed. Empathy creates conditions whereby both physicians and patients discover meaning. Empathy teaches that how physicians arrive at accurate medical diagnoses is just as important as getting there. The key to unlocking the power of empathy is not so much bringing empathy into medical practice, but keeping it there despite the rewards of technology and the tremendous advances in medical knowledge.

Case study: "Doc Peterson would be proud!"

In doing research for this book, I spent countless hours interviewing, observing and listening to physicians from all over the country. I ended up with volumes of data and relevant stories to assist in talking about the spirituality of medicine. One such interview took place during one of the breaks in the "Medicine in Search of Meaning" program. Sam P. is a practicing gastroenterologist, 46 years old, married, with three children. He is in practice with one other physician and, by his own admission, is enjoying the fruits of his labors – with one very looming exception.

Bill: Sam, you talked a lot today about what motivated you to go to medical school in the first place. You mentioned your uncle who was a pharmacist in rural Wisconsin and how you used to deliver medicines to patients of the two doctors that lived and worked in your hometown. You indicated that over time you gradually began to do odd jobs for them after school and on weekends. I think you said it was in your senior year of high school that you were asked to drive one of them around visiting patients who were homebound. What happened during that time that made you so adamant about going to medical school?

Sam: Doc Peterson was his name. He was a real character, warm, caring and very giving of his time and energy to all his patients. It was the way in which he truly listened to his patients' stories – even when they rambled on, telling him things that happened 50 years ago! Doc P. used to sit there and hold the hands of "his people," as he was fond of calling them. He was tired as hell one day ... I remember it was a Friday night just as the office was being closed. I was sweeping up his examination rooms when a call came in for him. I remember him taking a deep breath and closing his eyes just before he picked up the phone. He took Mrs. Simmons' call with all the attention and energy of his first patient that day. He seemed really there for her – focused, if you know what I mean. Doc P. asked me to drive him over to her house on the outskirts of town. On the way over, he told me that Mrs. Simmons was the very first patient he had some 30 years ago when he hung up his shingle. He told me she was in remarkably good health despite the arthritis that confined her to her home. When we got to her front door, he knocked and opened the door. I remember the wonderful aroma of homemade chicken soup that greeted us. Doc P. went over to her bedside and holding her hand, he remarked how wonderful she looked. He asked her about her family and the books she was reading. After listening attentively for about five minutes, he reached into his black bag and pulled out a few samples of cough medicine that he always seemed to have stashed away in there. Mrs. Simmons had a bad chest cold, sneezing and coughing. Even I knew she only had a cold. After eating a delicious bowl of chicken soup, Doc and I were back on the road again. On the way, I asked him why he didn't call the pharmacy and have a prescription delivered to her. Then something remarkable happened – he pulled the car over to the side of the road, put it in neutral, and told me to look him square in the eye. Of course I did. He said something to me that I haven't thought about in years. "Sam," he said, "if you eventually go on to medical school and become a doctor, I will get out of my grave and haunt you if you don't have the courage and interest to listen to the stories of your patients. Your future patients will be like beautifully wrapped gifts – you will never know what is inside until you take the time to unwrap them!" This was my first insight into what you are calling empathy.

Bill: It sounds like Doc Peterson's advice had a profound effect on you. How is it influencing you today in your current practice of medicine?

Sam: Doc P. died during my senior year of college. I went home for the funeral and I swear the whole county turned out for it. The last person I saw leaving the cemetery was Mrs. Simmons who waved at me. I walked over to her to see how she was doing. She told me that Doc P. would talk about me whenever he made his routine house calls to her home. She said that he looked upon me as his protege and was so proud that I was following in his footsteps. I remember standing there in the cemetery crying like a little baby when I heard that ... I think I'm avoiding your question ... I, um, well ... you see.... (Tears were welling up in Sam's eyes.)

Our conversation picked up later in the day after completion of the program. Sam sought me out and asked if I could stay on for a while. He had more to say.

Bill: You were really close to Doctor Peterson in your heart of hearts, weren't you Sam? Your tears told me there is still some unfinished business. Care to talk about it?

Sam: I really do.... All the way through medical school and well into my residency program, Doc P.'s influence was very conscious and evident in my life as an aspiring physician. Then things began to happen really fast and only this morning have I gotten in touch with them. At the end of my second year of residency, I got married. Six months later I was a proud father of a baby girl. Marge and I sat down one night before Gloria was born and in a near panic, realized the amount of debt we had incurred. A starter house, medical school bills, and a child on the way did not leave a lot to our imaginations. Reality was setting in. Marge was also in a residency program. We both wanted a big family, but knew that money would be tight for a long time. I think it was about that time that I started to think different thoughts about a future medical practice. Marge wanted to become a pathologist

– loving both the science aspects of that practice, as well as the normal hours of 9 to 5 so she could be home with the kids. It worked out well for her. I chose to shift from internal medicine to gastroenterology because it was of great interest to me and because of the earning potential that specialty had. Gradually, I began to think about my medical practice differently. Doc P. went to a quiet place inside, I think. Replacing him was the excitement I felt about the tremendous technological advances and knowledge base generated within my chosen specialty. Couple that with the normal rat race and treadmill life of a young doctor learning his craft and you can see what happened to me. As you described, Bill, my original dream was gone. Choosing gastroenterology was not the problem, it was not choosing to be more connected to my heart and dream. As I reflect upon the past dozen years, I can see that my mindset was changing. As one diagnostic challenge after another came my way ... as one child after another entered my life.... I guess I never really took time to think about what was inside of me. I was too busy taking care of others. Empathy was not part of my doctoring pattern. I hadn't even thought of Doc P. until you asked about the dreams that led me into medicine. Shit ... I bet old Doc P. is going to follow through on his threat to jump out of his grave and come after me!

Bill: He may have just done that today Sam. But not in the way you think. It is not too late you know. Maybe Doctor Peterson is carving out a spot for himself in your heart as we speak?

Before I left for home that Saturday, I sat in the hotel lobby and recorded my conversation with Sam while it was fresh in my mind. It was so powerful. What happens to the dreams that inspire us to greatness, that inspire us to integrate qualities like empathy, service, and active listening into our daily experiences? What factors in our life's journey allow those energizing dreams to be eroded and go to quiet places inside? By keeping empathy integrated into the diagnostic process, physicians can indeed "unwrap the beautiful gift that is each patient." Doctor Peterson would be proud.

Intangible benchmarks

There are defining moments when we clearly know the link between our soul's life and our capacity to be creative, productive and happy in our work. The human spirit has a dogged desire to discover a home in the world of work – a world of doing and having things, and of being in relationships. Financial success is not the only benchmark we have. Happiness, meaning, and a sense of well being are the intangible benchmarks that are present when the inner life of our soul is in sync with our activity in the outer world. However, what happens to us when our work becomes an authoritarian, all encompassing dominator of our existence? What happens when we lose balance, when success breeds, not happiness, but a malaise of boredom and lack of purpose?

Case study

I met Eric, a cardiovascular surgeon in his late forties, in his office to interview him for a book I am writing. On his wall is a picture of the Chinese symbol that means either problem or opportunity, depending on a person's state of mind. In America, we refer to seeing the glass of water as half–full or half–empty, depending on our outlook on life. Eric was talking with me about the intensity of his work and the need he has to hone his surgical skills and knowledge base on a continual basis. He acknowledged to me that he was "obsessive" about his study and research habits, as well as describing himself as a "perfectionist." I asked him about the meaning he placed on the Chinese symbol picture hanging on the wall. He said he found that picture at a rummage sale back when he was in his early years of residency. "I never wanted to be a physician who consistently had the attitude that life is a problem to be solved rather than an opportunity to be lived," he said. "Success had to mean more than being a great surgeon." I then asked him about where that thought is today in terms of his professional life. A long pause followed. Looking out the window to some distant spot on the horizon, he said, "Mine has been a calculating career that has desired success. I always wanted to be the best in whatever I did. I am achieving that goal (pause) but I feel kind of empty inside. Something seems to be missing. I had it once upon a time – that's why I was attracted to that Chinese symbol." Eric went on to talk about how he felt he had bailed out on taking care of himself in recent years by giving all his attention and creative energy to taking care of his practice. As we parted ways that day, Eric reflectively asked, "I wonder what ever happened to that hopeful, third year, surgical resident? Maybe I should dust off my picture and put it where I can see it with my heart again?"

Self-reflection

Are you in balance? The focus of our work is on cornering, regulating, and controlling our lives with concrete and well-defined goals. Our soul, on the other hand, discovers meaning and purpose, and hence pleasure, by letting go of control to the powers greater than human experience alone. What happens when your life gets out of whack – off center? How do you feel when you have mastered your work world and yet have a gnawing emptiness inside? How does it feel when you spend an inordinant amount of time reflecting on the deeper questions of your life and neglecting your work world? Stop and think for a moment: You go to work, but it is your soul that you put into it. If either part is missing, both seem to get lost.

Is your work a personal vocation? Reflect on the previous year and the events, people, and issues in your life. Have you experienced any value in your life higher than personal survival to which you have committed yourself? How would you describe the larger context of your life within which you place your work as a physician? What gifts do you bring to your world that will leave it a better place for your being there? Do your personal and professional talents suggest that being a physician is indeed a personal vocation?

Do you acknowledge? There is a marvelous and poignant short verse in the Hippocratic Oath that speaks to the vocation of being a physician: "Whatever house I enter, I shall come to heal." As we pay attention to what has heart and meaning for us, we will approach becoming a healer. Healers are people, physicians or not, who are skilled in the art of acknowledgment. As healers, physicians first acknowledge the power of their own inner spirit and bring that power and energy into their work and their relationship with their patients.

They acknowledge that heart and soul must be brought into the diagnostic process, into the use of medical technology, and into the skills they have honed over time. "Nemo dat quod non habit" – "I cannot give what I myself do not have."

Your Thoughts Along The Way

*(Take a moment to write down any thoughts
or insights you want to remember.)*

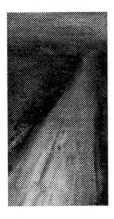

Chapter Nine

TAKING TIME TO BREATHE

"There is nothing busier than the ant,

yet it finds time to go to picnics"

A friend with wisdom in his heart once shared this thought with me during a time of change and distress in my life: "If any area of your life is not working, one of your beliefs in that area needs to be changed." A profoundly wonderful event prompted me to remember my friend's sage advice; my twin children, Sammy and Jessie, were born.

Picture this: it's 3:00 in the morning and both children are experiencing the promptings of nature, from both ends, I might add. At two months of age, there is very little sensitivity to the needs of mom and dad. I crawl out of bed rather reluctantly and grope for some dry diapers and milk bottles. By now I am doing this in my sleep. I tend to their needs and plop back into bed.

Now doing this once, twice, or even three times in one night is not too demanding. But this ritual had been going on for nearly eight weeks with no relief in sight. I was slowly becoming disenchanted with all those people who told me how wonderful fatherhood would be. Where were they at three o'clock in the morning preaching their good wishes? As the weeks came and went, I found myself becoming rather cranky, on edge, and falling asleep at my office. I prayed for the time when Sammy and Jessie and I would all sleep through the night. However, with no relief in sight, daddy got up several times each night and went through the usual routine. Then something rather remarkable happened.

It was about 4:30 a.m. and I had just finished putting the kids back to bed. I made a cup of coffee and was sitting at the kitchen table when my friend's thought came to me: "If one area of my life is not working (and this was one of those areas), one of my beliefs in that area needs to be changed." Now I don't have a clue why certain thoughts come to me when they do, but I am now a believer that I receive inspiration and meaning at the times I am most open and in need of them. This was one of those moments for me. A lesson was being born from within my own consciousness. Here is what I heard myself saying: "Bill, why do you think your children were given to you in the first place? For your convenience? I guess not. They were given to you so you could learn to love in ways that would only be possible if they were in your life. Examine your assumptions (beliefs) about what being a father is all about. Do you believe in your heart that you are meant to learn from them – that they are indeed your teachers?" I was being asked by my own inner teacher to examine my beliefs about being a father.

That quiet, reflective time sitting in the kitchen in the early morning was a real turning point for me. I realized that I was so busy "doing daddy stuff" that I was forgetting about the deeper meaning I could experience in "being a daddy." What does it mean to be a father and hence to do daddy stuff with a deeper sense of meaning and purpose? What lessons are Sammy and Jessie trying to teach me? These, and similar questions, began to flow out of that quiet, reflective time. Later in the day, I wrote this brief thought in my journal: "Learning the lessons that love has to offer is so often a retrospective experience. Yet, the lessons can help shape a new consciousness for the future." Because of this defining moment in my life, a major shift in consciousness began to occur within me. The next "three o'clock in the morning" experience would be my testing ground.

Sure enough, both Sammy and Jessie cooperated beautifully. They awoke, crying, hungry and ready for new diapers. Nothing at all changed externally. I was tired and they needed my attention. What had changed, however, was a deeper sense of meaning for my doing what I was going to do anyway. I brought a new mind set into an ordinary experience that I had repeated for weeks on end. The change was within me. The first thing I did upon entering their rooms was to greet them in a quiet, gentle and loving way. Unlike my old pattern of behavior, I brought something new to the experience. Instead of simply going through the functions of changing diapers and warming the bottles, I had a renewed sense of purpose for being there. They must have sensed something different about me, because neither child fussed as much as usual. They still cried until I changed and fed them. But I brought a new attitude and openness for learning to the encounter. My energy was different, and I believe that Sammy and Jessie picked it up, in their own little way. I began to believe with heart and soul that I could not change anyone – not really. All I can do is change myself and in so doing, my energy changes, and it calls out to the other for a different response. I cannot control how others respond to me. I can only change myself.

The way in is the way out: applications to medical practice.

When we experience conflicts or problems that need resolution, we have choices. One such choice is the "trial and error" method – do something different, try it and see if it works. If it doesn't, then try plan B. Sooner or later, something positive might happen. Sometimes, this method is effective in resolving disputes and disagreements with others, at least on the surface. We simply change our behavior and see if that satisfies the other party. For instance, let's say your neighbor does not like that fact that you mow your lawn at 7:00 on Saturday mornings. If the only thing you do when confronted with the issue by your neighbor is to mow the lawn at 10:00, you will have solved the problem – at least for your neighbor. But without a shift inside of you to freely change your mowing time, what might you begin to feel? Resentment? Frustration? Anger?

Changing for others will most likely meet their needs, but what about our needs? Even small changes done for the sake of appease-ment often lead to larger internal issues like resentment. With the trial and error method of behavior change, we change without a concurrent inner sense of knowing that we changed because this is the way we choose to respond to the situation. When we make a conscious choice to change in response to situations, rather than just reacting, we stay grounded in our own center of power; with the trial and error method, we remain grounded in the power of another. Our personal power consists of our capacity to choose how we respond to situations that our life presents – no matter how seemingly small and insignificant. Meaning and purpose then become by–products of that kind of deci-sion–making.

A case study

Dr. Jon T. is a primary care physician employed by a hospital locat-ed in a rather large urban area. This hospital has entered into a sub-stantial managed care contract with a large health insurance company. The majority of Jon's patients are the people covered by this carrier. Part of his compensation is tied into his ability to manage resources. Utilization management is a key component to his economic well being. One other factor important to note – Jon is a very ethical and moral person. I got a sense of this during my time with him and also by some comments made by his peers.

The case study begins with Jon receiving 7:30 a.m. telephone calls from the hospital's utilization manager. Over a period of three months, the utilization manager tells Jon he needs to be more "discriminating" with his hospital admissions and specialty referrals. These fairly con-stant communications began to irk Jon, but as a "dutiful doctor" (his own words), he began to examine and change his referral and admis-sion frequency. There were even times he felt it was to the detriment of full patient care as he judged it. Using the "trial and error" method, he changed and complied because of outside pressures. However, he did not feel good about it in his heart. Over time, his resentment grew towards managed care, the utilization manager, and hospital and physi-cian leaders. Jon was fast becoming known as a disgruntled camper. When I initially interviewed him, the second sentence out of Jon's mouth was: "Nuts to this shit. Nobody is going to tell me how to care for my patients."

Towards the end of a lengthy conversation with him, I suggested that Jon try another way – one that would take both the demands of the other (in this case the managed care system), and Jon's energies and competencies into consideration. I call this method "the way in is the way out." This method allows us to remain grounded in our soul – a soul that brings power and energy to the situation. We make choices and changes out of inner strength, not external compliance alone. It works this way: demands or requests are made of us, however we choose to frame it for ourselves. In the external scheme of things only (the trial and error method), we have three options. One, we can comply with the demand; two, we do not comply with the demand; or three, we can argue until the cows come home for the demand to be rescinded. We usually try the third option, but to little or no avail in the long run. Then we fall back on options one or two. Choosing any option in this scenario, we will eventually become disgruntled campers unless something internal begins to happen for us. That something internal is the sense of meaning or purpose that we bring to the situation. Our internal reason or meaning for whether we accept the demand and act on it is ours alone. We take the demand inside and begin to ask questions like – What is this experience asking of me? How can I make sense out of it for me? What is the bigger picture that I may not be seeing clearly? The experience of the demand can actually become a teachable moment for us, requiring us to bring our soul life forward in a conscious way. Whatever internal response we discover ultimately, our soul guides our decision making and our subsequent behavior. No one else can do that for us; nor can they take that power away from us. Only we can surrender our power, that is, give it up in mere external compliance to a demand from another. Meaning for our choices or mandated behavior must come from within or else something gets lost in the shuffle. The consequence of choosing not to bring meaning and purpose to a situation is anger, resentment, and even bitterness. By accessing our own inner world of meaning, we can bring another level of awareness to what we choose to do and to what we are asked to do.

In Jon's case, I encouraged him to ask questions like "What does it mean for me to practice medicine in a managed care setting?" and "What does it mean for me to bring my own power of choice to bear on a utilization demand?" These reflective questions are Jon's "way in" to the choices he will have to make. His "way out" is the concrete sense of meaning (his own internal reasons) that will emerge, that is, his own personal response. By bringing the issue inside for personal discovery of meaning, he will maintain his own identity and internal freedom as a practicing physician without the baggage of anger, resentment, or growing bitterness. He may have to walk with the questions for awhile, but sooner, rather than later, a meaningful response will come into his consciousness – a response that will make sense to him.

Many times, whether we like it or not, our choices are limited in the external world. Death, taxes, washing the dishes, food shopping, and changing diapers for our children are but a few examples of those external limitations on our freedom. However, our internal choices that move us closer towards meaning and purpose, are never limited by external factors. How we process our questions, how we internally handle the demands of our world – these are ours and ours alone. To surrender to them is to become a slave; to respond internally is to be free. "What is this experience trying to teach me?" becomes a critical question. No one has power over the way we think about, or process, a given situation or demand. By reclaiming our birthright, our heritage, our power, we will have the capacity to discover meaning and purpose in even the smallest of events or the most trivial of demands.

I can still picture Jon sitting across from me, coffee cup in hand and eyes wide open, saying: "So what you are suggesting, Bill, is that if I stay angry or resentful toward a person or system, it is my fault ultimately? ... that blame is simply a part of my personality's bag of tricks to keep me grounded in anger and resentment? ... that it is ultimately my lack of responding internally to the demands of my life that causes so much distress?" Nodding positively to his insightful observations, I encouraged him to be aware that this dynamic of blame, which can play out in very subtle ways. Only my ego knows the defense mechanism of blame; my soul does not.

Breathing moments

Breathing moments, or brief moments of time wherein we hold our life still, are the key to unlocking the power of our soul and bringing its energy into the experiences of our life. I am not suggesting using breathing moments to gain control over our life; but rather to live more deeply into our life's questions. In the clinical practice of medicine – in fact, in the current culture of medicine today – we find a world moving towards scientific surety, technological advancement, and diagnostic breakthroughs. This world is characterized by medical practitioners honing their rational and deliberative skills, with the end product being the conquering of disease and illness. This predominantly left brain activity has done wonders for the advancements in medical science that are available to the clinical practitioner. What is missing, I believe, is the right brain activity of the poet, the reflective thinker, the creator, the healer, and the discoverer of meaning. Imagine, for a moment, a bridge connecting the left side of your brain (the logical, rational, scientific side) with the right side of your brain (the healing, creative, affective, and spiritual side). Furthermore, imagine a midpoint on that bridge with a severe break in it that does not allow easy access from one side to the other. By allowing ourselves breathing moments, we can literally reconnect both sides and see them as valuable resources. In times of need, we can breathe deeply, hold our life still, and travel to soulful, meaningful side of our life. We can bring the demands, problems, and related issues that need the attention to the right side of our brain. Each experience of our life, then, can become an opportunity for new growth and learning. We will no longer need blame, rationalizations, and the like to shield us from feeling and experiencing our life situations. By utilizing "the way in is the way out" strategy, each day's demands and opportunities can become a more intimate way of staying connected to our own spiritual path and the creative energies that are at the core of who we are. Jon left our conversation with this thought: "Maybe my life's thirst for meaning can be quenched even in the midst of the most mundane demands of my practice? It was me who really gave power to the managed care system by not learning to access my own."

Perhaps we do give power to what we pay attention to?

The time will come when, with elation, you will greet yourself arriving at your own door, in your own mirror, and each will smile at the other's welcome and say, sit here. Eat. You will love again the stranger who was yourself. Give wine. Give bread. Give back your heart to itself, to the stranger who has loved you all your life, whom you ignored for another, who knows you by heart.

—Derek Walcott, from his book *Sea Grapes*

Case Study

While participating in a recent clinical conference, a general surgeon I knew approached me looking a bit frazzled. I asked him how he was doing and all he kept repeating was: "My wife and kids just don't understand what I am about!" After repeating this mantra at least three times, I sensed he was getting perturbed, even angry, at their perceived "lack of sensitivity to the demands of my medical practice." During a break in the conference, John asked me for a few moments to talk privately about what was occurring in his life.

John is a busy and successful general surgeon. Referrals are plentiful because of his skill and expertise. He is married, with three children ranging from ages 9 to 17. John has been in practice for 14 years. To keep up his knowledge and practice of new technologies and procedures, John has frequently been away from his family to participate in ongoing medical education. During our conversation, I asked him to describe his experiences as a general surgeon, particularly any defining moments for him. The first thing out of his mouth was: "When I'm practicing my craft, I am the captain of the ship. I speak and people get me what I need." I asked John if he carries that attitude over into his personal life. He immediately denied that he did. I asked him to reflect for a moment on the issue of balance between his personal and professional life – not in terms of equality of time and energy, but in terms of quality time and energy. His response: "I think I bring home my physician hat every day I do surgery. Thinking about it now, maybe I expect my family to treat me like my surgical team does – captain of the ship!" Before returning to the clinical conference, John looked at me and said: "Perhaps I am the cause of my frustration with my wife and kids. When I go home, I think I expect every one else's life to stop and focus on what I need. Am I that egocentric that I expect the world to revolve around me?" I shook John's hand and congratulated him on beginning his path to wisdom.

Self–reflection

Do you balance doing and being? To define ourselves rather exclusively by what we do is to buy into a culture that prizes doing over being – that values work over cultivating the life of the soul. As in most of life, the issue isn't "either ... or" but "both ... and" – not one thing over another, but one thing and another. The key to enhancing the quality of our life, and consequently a sense of hopefulness, rests squarely in developing balance: a balance between family and work, work and self–care. To know we are rooted in our spiritual path is to come to know balance as a friend. We need to pay quality time, energy, and conscious attention to the balancing act in which we often find ourselves. What area of your life is not working right now? Where do you experience the most frustration? the deepest depression? the most anxiety? What part of your life are you ignoring? These kinds of questions will lead us to discover deeper meaning and purpose in whatever we are about.

Do you cultivate your spirit? I read this somewhere: "A soul met an angel and asked: 'By which path shall I reach heaven quickest – the path of knowledge or the path of love?' The angel looked wonderingly and said: 'Are not both paths one?' " A physician friend of mine observed that his training prepared him excellently for doing medicine, but woefully lacked a value being placed on heart, mind and spiritual growth. He went on further to share this rather profound insight: "If I could change any one thing about the culture of medicine in this country, it would be to teach medical students and physicians to think as an individual person with heart, mind and spirit, not exclusively as an objective professor or clinician." What have you done lately to cultivate the powers of your own inner spirit? Have you taken quality time to simply hold your life still for awhile and to allow your heart to feel what it needs to feel? What is your life asking of you today? Where is balance most needed? To whom do you need show appreciation and thanks?

To what are you attached? We can uncover where our life is out of balance by looking at our attachments. Attachments are specific, immovable expectations, and desires that are projected onto people, places, and situations in our life. Wherever we are unduly attached is where we will become controlling and rigid. If this thought makes sense, then it makes even greater sense to look at the experience of detachment, that is, our capacity to calmly observe our reactions to situations and people and to not get pulled into an emotional position. When we can do this in the area where our life is most out of balance (in John's case with his medical practice), then it stands to reason that we can make choices for change. Practicing medicine can be as addictive a behavior as drinking and using drugs. When work is addictive, our life gets out of balance. When our life is out of balance, we tend to get defensive and go into denial mode. Frustration and anger become partners in blaming others for "not being sensitive to me and what I am about." John knows what I mean.

Your Thoughts Along The Way

*(Take a moment to write down any thoughts
or insights you want to remember.)*

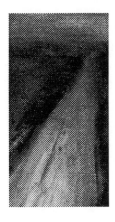

Chapter Ten

WHEN DOCTORS
BECOME PHYSICIANS

In each of our lives, no matter what our profession, we have experienced specific and undeniable defining moments that give form and substance to our life and our work. Defining moments (experiences) are not chosen as such. They present themselves as lessons to be learned – as opportunities to be seized. They just happen, very much like surprises. For our purposes, defining moments are intimate, challenging, personal responses to seemingly innocent interactions with self, others, and/or the environment. Seldom are they big issues or events. On the contrary, they are deeply personal responses to small events that make it possible for the larger events to happen. Defining moments have the capacity to change the course of a life, impacting vocational, relational, and professional choices. They arrive when they are least expected. But something inside us is touched off by that momentary experience. In a defining experience, a conscious, "aha" moment occurs that somehow touches the very core of who we are. Our soul is stirred.

This seemingly small experience, then, has the potential to lead to an even deeper examination of our life – or some aspect of our life, like our work. An internal connection to a sense of personal meaning begins to germinate, causing us to rethink some of our beliefs, values, behaviors, and/or previous choices. An internal, affective, and moving experience begins to happen with ever widening circles of influence. Picture a pebble being tossed in the middle of a clear, calm pool of water. The entry point becomes the defining moment. The ripples that go out from that entry point are the influences that have the capacity to lead us towards change of some sort. They become the provocative stirrings of our soul calling us to reassessment. I remember writing the following thought in my journal after a defining moment for me: "Something is happening to me – I'm not sure what it is right now. All I can say is I sense that some dimension of my life needs to change ... my perception of reality is different. I find myself being affected more deeply than I thought. What I know is simply this: something is stirring inside that I sense will have a profound influence on what I do from now on."

Defining moments are not always perceived initially as positive experiences. They might even be painful at the time, causing some distress, anxiety, or even anger. Whatever the case, the ramifications of that initial experience may not present themselves in their entirety all at once. We need self–reflection; holding our life still for awhile so that we might consciously accept the fact that this experience is indeed trying to teach us something that will become a sine qua non.

I remember a conversation I had with a family medicine, third–year resident named Pam. I was interviewing her while doing research for this book. We met right after morning report where she was coming off of a 12–hour shift. To say that she was tired would be an understatement. During morning report, Pam presented a complicated case she was assigned during the night. I do not remember all the details, but at one point during her presentation, a staff physician challenged her rather strongly about the diagnosis she had arrived at. I could see this young resident starting to lose it, becoming angry and frustrated. Fortunately, the staff physician backed off and the case discussion went on. As she and I sat together in the hospital dining room having coffee, she was clearly not in a great mood. After talking a bit about what she was feeling, Pam apologized for being so tired. "No need to apologize," I said. "Why don't we set another time for this interview?" She agreed. "But before you go, Pam, take this question with you – what is this experience trying to teach you? We can talk about your response next week." Pam said she would do that.

A week went by, and as I sat in the hospital dining room waiting for Pam, I wondered which Pam would be here for our meeting – the tired, exhausted, and frustrated Pam or a calmer version. As she approached the table, I saw a smiling young woman whose eyes were alive. Before she even sat down, Pam said to me: "Bill, I want to thank you. After I woke up last week, I began to think about the question you posed and decided that it was stupid and irrelevant. Three days later, I still found myself angry with that staff physician. It was bugging me to no end. So I said to myself, 'Pam, as a last resort, maybe you should think about the question. What do you have to lose?' So I did spend some time thinking about what that experience was trying to teach me. Nothing really came to me until this morning. All of a sudden, I had this thought in relationship to my experience last week – maybe I need to take better care of myself so I can fulfill the demands of practicing medicine."

"Wonderful, Pam. It sounds like you have made sense out of what happened to you last week in a way that can really serve your life – especially your future medical practice. Allow this response to grow and follow through on your insight of taking care of yourself. How do you feel about the physician who confronted you?"

"I don't feel angry. In fact, and this sounds crazy, but I am almost grateful for the experience."

Because Pam was open to learning from her encounter that morning, it became a defining moment for her. All defining moments are retrospective in nature. By allowing ourselves some quiet, internal space to process and ask questions of ourselves, we can empower experiences to serve us rather profoundly. Self–dialogue has the power to awaken our curiosity around making sense out of whatever happens – whether it is perceived positively or negatively. A great metaphor for this process of allowing defining moments to emerge can be a fly buzzing around our head. It just will not go away no matter how many times we swat at it with our hands. In fact, it seems to gain steam and become even more bothersome. But the moment we get still and do not move, it will land soon enough. It, too, becomes still. We can then figure out what we want to do about it being there.

A case study: my personal, defining moment

No one on God's good earth can tell us when a defining experience will occur for us. Only we can allow that to happen. The experience becomes defining for us when in retrospect, we say it is so and make it so. The meaning and purpose that we uncover over time as a by–product of reflection gives it the defining label. Even though the experience itself may, by external standards, be micro in nature, we alone allow internal meaning connections to surface, impacting the macro world of our life and our work.

One such moment occurred for me when I heard the news of Dr. Harold Borkawf's death. I picked up the telephone at home around 4:45 p.m. on Friday, February 23, 1995. My friend, Len Scarpinato, Harold's personal physician, who was on call that day, informed me about the bad news and some of the details surrounding his untimely death. As I shared the news with Peg, I kept thinking "why did this have to happen to such a wonderful and caring person?"

Harold's heart was kept going through life support systems. Essentially, all brain functioning had ceased. There was nothing that could pull him through the ravages of a ruptured, cerebral aneurism. A sinking feeling – a helpless feeling – overpowered me as I left for the hospital. I reminisced over the experiences I had with Harold – the birth of Sammy and Jessie, the humorous banter he always seemed to carry on with Peg, the most current books he was reading. I even remembered the time I looked into his car and saw a mini library growing in the back seat. Upon arrival at the hospital, I stopped at the administration offices to see my friend, Sister Renee Rose, St. Mary's Hospital president. We sat in her office for awhile sharing stories about Harold. Tears welled up in our eyes as we fondly recalled what he meant to each of us.

I dreaded going over to the Intensive Care Unit. On my way over there, I paused briefly in the hospital lobby to catch my breath. It was there, in a breath–taking moment in the hospital's lobby, that a specific visit with Harold came crashing into my awareness. He was sitting behind his office desk talking with Peg and I about the impending birth of our children. He was laughing and joking with Peg to put her at ease. With a wink in my direction, he looked solemnly at Peg and proceeded to tell her to stay in bed for the remainder of the pregnancy to avoid potential complications. "Don't worry, Margaret," he said, "if I could take away your pain and discomfort, I would. You will be just fine. In a few weeks you will have two beautiful babies to hold in your arms." We all chuckled and Harold gave Peg a hug as we left for home.

Why this experience with Harold came to mind, I do not know. What I do know is that he gave us more than a doctor's relationship with a patient. His sense of humor always seemed to come to the fore-front, especially in difficult times during the pregnancy. Humor was his way of gently caring for people. Harold was always present to us – made us feel special – as if we were his only patients. That was the image of him that stuck in my mind's eye, standing there in the lobby. As I arrived at the elevator, I knew in a flash that I would write this book and dedicate it to Harold. Before that moment, I talked about writing, but did little or nothing to actually do it. His death turned into a defining, motivating moment for me. The next day I turned on my computer. To this very day, I thank Harold for all that he continues to mean to me and my family.

A metaphor: doctor or physician?

Webster's New World Dictionary defines the word metaphor as "a figure of speech in which one thing is spoken of as if it were another." A metaphor can become very abstract and subtle when used to present an idea to others. It has the power to add a richness and depth to the idea in hopes of revealing meanings that are not readily apparent. Metaphors are descriptive words used to convey those meanings in a succinct way. They need to be reflected upon for those meanings to surface. For example, a metaphor is like an onion, with layers that need to be peeled back to reveal deeper layers of meaning – or a gift that needs to be unwrapped before it can be enjoyed.

I have met, experienced, and known many, many doctors over the years. Not all of them were physicians. Let me explain.

Doctors are wonderfully intelligent, gifted people who have developed great skills, diagnostic capacities, and a wide body of scientific knowledge. They clearly know how to treat people, help maintain quality of life, and apply and prescribe a wide array of technological advancements and pharmaceutical treatments. Doctors become doctors when they complete a demanding and rigorous training process and become certified to practice medicine. That is what is required to become a doctor. Doctors apply what they have learned from medical experience to their patients. A doctor, metaphorically speaking, is a word used to describe a unilaterally powerful person who has trained for years to do something for others and to others. Essentially, a doctor practices medicine on a one–way street that is characterized by a giving only – a giving out of his or her vast storehouse of knowledge and experience. It is a one–way relationship. Giving to patients is not a bad thing; however, if that is all that happens, it is a limiting experience for the doctor and the patient.

Physicians, on the other hand, are people who can do all of the above, but do it in a relationally powerful way. Unlike a doctor who focuses on dispensing knowledge and skills to the patient, a physician is a person who has developed the gift of being open to new insights and knowledge on a human, spiritual level. Physicians bring their humanness, their own inner spirits, to their practice of medicine. They have a conscious investment in their own spiritual growth, and bring that dimension, along with their medical expertise, to their practice. Physicians are open to learning – to defining moments. They do not, for example, get so immersed in their practices that they forget the art of self–reflection, the need for self–care, and their general, overall personal quality of life. In a nutshell, they do not simply identify themselves solely in their roles as doctors. Physicians realize they have an inner life and they have learned to nurture that life.

As physicians remain open to defining moments in every facet of their lives, personal and professional, the human dimension of their medical practices does not go unnoticed or unattended. Through a basic openness to others, physicians cultivate the art of listening with more than their ears; they learn what caring and empathy are all about, especially when their medical skills are not enough. Physicians know the art of healing, not just treating and curing. They practice medicine on a two–way street that is characterized by both giving and receiving, influencing as well as being influenced. Physicians practice medicine with their patients; doctors practice medicine on their patients. Perhaps not all doctors have learned the art of being a physician?

A case study

A 61–year–old woman named Mary came into a clinic after she had fallen on the sidewalk outside of her apartment complex. Her presenting complaints to a second–year resident, Mac, who was on clinic rotation, were: extreme soreness in her shoulder and arm, as well as two lacerations on her arm caused by falling on glass. Mac treated her lacerations and ordered an X–ray on her arm and shoulder. They came back negative. Just as Mac was finishing up, a nurse brought in a copy of her medical history. Mary had been an inpatient at the adjoining hospital as well an outpatient on several occasions. Her medical history included a radical mastectomy on both her breasts (age 47) as well a mild heart attack (age 59). Mary also suffered from an acute arthritic condition and was under a specialist's care. She was in almost constant pain and discomfort. Other facts about Mary: she lived alone in a one room apartment two blocks from the hospital. She didn't get out much due to her arthritis. She had no immediate family members in the area, but had several friends who lived in the same apartment complex. Before she left for home in the clinic van, Mary turned to Mac and said: "You are such a wonderful and kind person, having taken such good care of me. Won't you please come over to my home for cookies and milk!" Mary's eyes sparkled as she patted Mac's hand.

Little did Mac know then, but he was being invited into a defining moment both personally and professionally. He couldn't get Mary out of his mind even while he saw a steady stream of clinic patients that afternoon. He was struck deeply by the warmth of Mary's presence and charm. Here was a person who had every reason to be bitter and angry, to feel lonely and cut off, and most certainly to lack any sense of meaning and purpose in life.

The next day during the morning report, Mac spoke to the attending physician at the clinic about this experience with Mary – how she touched him with the simplicity and openness of her spirit. The attending simply challenged Mac: "What do you want to do about what you experienced yesterday?" After the morning report, Mac headed back to the clinic. He just knew that he needed to respond to the attending's question. He knew, deep down, that Mary's presence would be an important moment for him personally as well as professionally. "After all," Mac said, "aren't the Mary's of this world part of the reason I got into medicine in the first place?"

During his lunch break, Mac called Mary to inquire about stopping over after clinic to visit and check up on her pain medication. At 3:30 he rang her doorbell and was buzzed in. He wasn't ready for what he was to experience – a defining moment for sure!

Mary's small apartment was truly a home – clean and neat as a pin with a view of a park. Mac was greeted by Mary, sat down, and waited while Mary got the milk and cookies she promised! Sitting there, Mac saw how gingerly Mary walked, grimacing in pain. He was moved by the beautiful way she served him, treating him as if he were the only person on the planet. Tears welled up in Mac's eyes as he thought: "All my knowledge, skill and diagnostic expertise seem minuscule with what my heart is feeling." Mac ate his cookies, finished his milk and after a brief visit, left for home. The next morning, Mac found out that Mary had died that night of a massive heart attack. He attended her funeral and cried.

Now, a 48–year–old physician, practicing internal medicine with a sub–specialty in cardiology, Mac credits Mary with teaching him what he needed to learn about being a physician. To use his words, "I am now a physician, not just a doctor. My defining moment with Mary helped me in caring, healing and loving – all qualities of a physician. Coupled with my training, skill development and scientific knowledge, Mary and I make a wonderful team!" By taking some reflective time, Mac turned a clinic moment into a physician/patient encounter influencing the direction of his life.

Self–Reflection

Are you learning from your defining moments? What are possible defining moments for you – experiences just waiting to help shape who you are? Have you lost the impact and force of past defining moments? If so, how will you continue to learn from them, to reconnect with their power? What is your vocation as a physician asking of you today? Where are the "Mary" experiences in your life? Can you allow them to give form and substance to your clinical practice of medicine?

Our enthusiasm for what we do can be affected by not being open to defining moments.

"Age may wrinkle my face,
but lack of enthusiasm will wrinkle my soul!"

Your Thoughts Along The Way

*(Take a moment to write down any thoughts
or insights you want to remember.)*

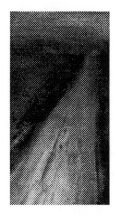

Chapter Eleven

WHERE IN GOD'S NAME AM I?

What does it mean to wake up and live more deeply into our life? What are the implications of seeing our life primarily through the eyes of other people and not our own? When, exactly, does our spiritual journey start? How long have we been strangers to the life of our own soul and its promptings? Fresh questions will come, replacing the worn out, standard responses to life to which we have grown accustomed. Fresh questions came to me as I reflected on the following Native American story as told in the poet David Whyte's book The Heart Aroused (New York: Doubleday Books, 1994, pp. 259–260). Listen...

> *Stand still.*
> *The trees ahead and the bushes beside you*
> *Are not lost.*
> *Wherever you are is called Here,*
> *And you must treat it as a powerful stranger,*
> *Must ask permission to know it and be known.*
> *The forest breathes.*
> *Listen.*
> *It answers,*
> *I have made this place around you,*
> *If you leave it you may come back again, saying Here.*
> *No two trees are the same to Raven.*
> *No two branches are the same to Wren.*
> *If what a tree or a bush does is lost on you,*
> *You are surely lost.*

Stand still.
The forest knows Where you are.
You must let it find you.

I first heard this poem read aloud by David Whyte at a conference for Catholic health care leaders. It struck many deep cords inside of me. Actually, the truth be known, I was experiencing some anxiety as I listened intently. I was not altogether certain I wanted to be shaken from the comfortable perch I called my life. (Poetry has that affect on me – it gets my reflective processes headed in the direction of my soul. When that happens, I know I am being called to some kind of change.) One of those soul–related cords that came to me was in the form of a question: "Am I more concerned about making a good living than about how to live?" Why that particular question came to me, I do not know. I am learning, however, to observe and pay close attention to anything that pricks my soul.

Several questions began to emerge into consciousness. How, in fact, do I live? What gives primary meaning to me as I walk through my day? Who are my teachers and why do I get angry at them from time to time? And then this question surfaced: "Where is my wealth?" I knew I was being challenged to open up that question. As is becoming my custom, I reflected upon the metaphor of "wealth" as it related to meaning and purpose in my life. Wealth always signified what I was able to accumulate in terms of stocks, bonds, savings, and retirement nest eggs. This notion was extended to include owning a home, being secure financially with a good job, and being a parent to my children, Sammy and Jessie. I guess I always assumed I was a "wealthy" person relatively speaking. I never have had a lot of financial security, but always enough to provide for the needs of my family and myself. What was pricking my spirit was the notion that I was forgetting what real wealth was all about – a wealth that could never be taken away unless I allowed it to happen.

I was being challenged to view my wealth in very radical ways, ways that my personality or ego did not like. Slowly, but surely, my consciousness of wealth was being expanded to include not always knowing the outcome, taking risks, not trying to control others or events, a deep acceptance of my gifts to the world, an awareness of being called by a loving and forgiving God to become a co–creator, and last, but not least, the varied experiences I was presented with each and every day. I knew in my heart that my wealth was certainly more than I could accumulate. My wealth was expanded to include the people, events, and experiences life offers me. The choices I make in responding to this wealth make me who I am. It is this wealth that provides the underbedding to my life – it is what I bring to each encounter, every patient I see, each of my children, and each significant other in my life.

We invest in the wealth of our soul by being open to defining moments in our life, observing and being okay with our feelings at any given moment, dreaming about a more loving and sacred future rather than a blaming, fearful and profane one.

Recently, while reviewing my presentation notes for a conference for a group of physicians, I noted a conversation that I had with Jim. Jim was a 46–year–old cardiologist, married, with one child. Jim's journey to discover his wealth strongly paralleled mine, and perhaps yours. What follows is an account of the beginning of his journey as related to me during a late night conversation following the conference.

Jim: You challenged me, Bill, and I am not sure I liked it. I found myself getting angry with you for raising questions that I initially thought of as dumb and irrelevant. I was convincing myself that this conference was a waste of my time. My pager was all set to go off – if you know what I mean – and then you asked us the question about how we define ourselves, by our roles as provider, father/mother, doctor, husband/wife, and friend, or by who we are inside. I know both are important, but it was the second one, defining myself by who I am on the inside, that pulled my finger off the pager. You challenged us to go deeper into our lives, beneath the roles we are in. That's really hard for me to do because that's all I really know. I have invested a hell of a lot of time, money, and energy into those roles since the beginning of medical school. I don't know much about going any deeper into my life, beneath the roles I play. I pretty much define myself by what I do, by the roles, if you know what I mean. Nothing more, nothing less. Does that make any sense to you at all Bill?

Bill: It sure does, Jim. You are describing my spiritual journey to a tee! We are a lot alike. Let me ask you a question that challenged some time ago. Maybe it will help open some things up for you? Are you more concerned about making a good living than about how to live? This is not an either/or question, but a both/and one. What do you think? Where is your wealth, Jim?

Jim: That a hard question for me to respond to. I really don't think at all about how I live my life and how I take care of myself. I just do what I need to do, not a whole lot of reflection. What frightens me about the questions you ask is the feeling that my life is indeed out of balance, if you want to know the truth. In fact, in many ways it is out of control. I keep working hard because then I won't have to worry about feeling what I'm feeling. I know I put in long hours at work because that is what I know best. My wife and I get into arguments about my working such crazy and long hours. The more we argue, the more I work to avoid dealing with my part in the relationship. I also feel like I am on a treadmill in the office. I don't particularly like what I'm doing these days, it's kind of routine and boring. But I keep on plugging away, hoping that I'll feel something good one of these days.

Bill: And what are you feeling these days, Jim?

Jim: Like shit if you really want to know. I don't know where I am anymore like I once did. I think I am afraid to step back and to see what is really under the roles I play every day. I don't think there is much there. I really hate this empty, shitty feeling inside. I don't like doing this much thinking. In fact, I avoid it when possible. (The tone of Jim's voice was turning angry and harsh as he began to confront the inner wealth to which he has paid little attention over the years.)

Bill: Why don't you try something, Jim, that might help? Take a few sheets of paper and begin talking with yourself about what you are thinking and feeling about the real you underneath the roles. Don't worry about how you say it, just say it in writing as it comes to you. For starters, on top of the first page, write this sentence as many times as you need to in order to believe it: I am exactly where I need to be in my life right now. Whatever comes to mind, write it down. You don't have to show this journal to anyone. The reason for doing it is to shake things up inside, kind of like shaking the orange juice in the morning before drinking it. There are things that will come to you that need the light of day. Don't put a value judgment on what comes to you. Just let it flow like a stream of consciousness. Everything you say to yourself is what needs to be said. If you would like, why don't we have breakfast together tomorrow morning. We can talk about your new experience of yourself. (Jim agreed.)

While there is more to Jim's story than I am able to share, several important, life–giving things surfaced for him during his writing that night. When we met in the corner of the hotel's cafeteria for breakfast, Jim looked tired, but had a clearly perceived new look about him. The tone of his voice was much more gentle and sure of itself. He described himself that morning as "having a weight lifted off his spirit, his soul, and has allowed some very positive energy to surface inside." As Jim and I conversed, he was becoming more forgiving of himself, clearer about who he was and what he had been denying for years and years. Towards the end of our conversation that morning, Jim shared that he is less afraid now of what he is feeling, that there are indeed issues he needs to work on, but that this work would now be seen in the context of his wealth, and not his deprivation. Both of us acknowledged our time together as being defining moments – each in our own way deriving a new sense of meaning about who we were. As we were paying the bill for breakfast, Jim turned to me and said, "Thanks for showing me, for encouraging me, to accept the fact that I was on a spiritual journey for my whole life. The difference now is that I know I am on it and can take the time to consciously be without fear and to take better care of myself." As I walked to my car, I thought of how grateful I am to a God, a Divine Source of Life, who connects with us at times we can least imagine.

An inner dialogue between my soul and personality

At the same time Jim was talking to himself that night, I took the time to talk to myself.

Tell me my friend, just how are you defining yourself today? By your roles as father, provider, friend, writer, or by who you are inside that provides meaning and roots to what you do? You know, don't you, that your true identity is written and embossed in the very center of your being. This is your primary source of meaning that can never be taken away. In your roles, you can clearly see important sources of meaning, a source of meaning that is passing, even secondary. Why don't you pay attention to your primary source of meaning in balance with the secondary sources? Are you afraid of what you will discover? Perhaps. It's easier to look outside. Think of this for a moment: what is it that gives energy and meaning to what you do, to your roles in life? Where is love generated and expressed if not in and through your soul moving outward into all you do? Here is a new thought for your personality to consider: how does your personality feel about allowing me, your soul, out into every nook and cranny of your world? I think you know that your work, for example, will lose something if retreat to a quiet place inside. You get into trouble, Bill, when you forget about me altogether, or when things get so out of whack that you have no place else to turn except me. Now that's ok with me, but don't you think that if I were given the time and reflective attention that you, let's say, give to your work or worrying about the future, I would be in a better position to be your friend? The choice is yours to make or not to make. Just know that you have a choice.

Perhaps we can redeem any moment of our life by holding up and honoring all that life presents to us in the form of lessons to be learned, especially the wealth of that which is rejected and unwanted in our experiences.

An important case study

Harvey K. is a 51–year–old practicing physician in the field of family and community medicine. He is also the elected president of the medical staff. Divorced, and the father of three college–age children, his life is focused almost entirely on his work. Several important issues are impacting Harvey's life: 1) He is being called upon to lead a bitterly divided medical staff in ongoing negotiations with the local integrated health system on moving from autonomous, independent group practices to employment by the system; 2) Harvey's divorce was bitterly and angrily contested by his ex–wife, leaving him financially strapped and depressed; 3) Harvey's children blame him for the breakup of the marriage; and 4) Harvey's practice continues to grow, placing even more demands on his time and energy. One evening during a negotiations meeting, Harvey blew up and angrily denounced the attorneys representing both sides. He felt they were the only ones getting rich over these negotiations. After that meeting, Harvey stopped at a bar for his usual martinis and a bite to eat. He was stopped by the police and ticketed for drunken driving. After posting bail, he went home and contemplated suicide.

After listening to Harvey's story, I could not help but reconnect with some important lessons in my own life's journey. What do I do when my life's experiences just seem to come down upon me like a thrashing rain storm, with no relief in sight? How do I handle those difficult moments? What choices come to me? Crazy ones? Irrational ones that almost sound sane because they would relieve me of what I was feeling? One thing I have learned, and one that Harvey came to know and understand, is that we must accept ourselves where we are at any given moment. Accepting ourselves means learning to listen to and observe what we are feeling and thinking, pretty much as if we were a third party in our mind's eye observing the swirl of emotion overtaking us. When we can observe ourselves, we create an arm's length distance that allows us to catch our breath and quietly listen without judgment. When we hold up and honor our feelings in this way, we can then repeat this mantra over and over again: I am exactly where I need to be in my life right now. After we have said it enough that we begin to believe it (which we ultimately must if we want to move on and learn from this experience), then we are getting closer to allowing the following question to our best teacher: what is this experience trying to teach me? If we do not confront the real stuff of our life, and run away from what we are feeling by rationalizing and denying, we will only dig ourselves an even deeper hole.

Once we have truly accepted the fact that we are exactly where we need to be, then we are in a wonderful position to learn from our experiences, and to see that the unwanted parts of our life are in reality magnificent opportunities for growth and change. This is as much a part of our wealth as any savings account or investments. Our wealth, as Harvey and I have come to learn, is found in that which we so desperately want to reject and deny, or rationalize away. Our challenge is to make friends with what we usually reject, with what we see as bad or causing us grief and anger. Our ego or personality wants the "bad" to go away and will use any means to make that happen – blame, denial, rationalization, and projection. These defense mechanisms quite literally keep our soul from interacting with our lived experiences. The dark side of our ego has the tendency to make our world smaller by focusing on control and judgment. When this occurs, our soul retreats to a very quiet place inside.

The starting point

The starting point for growing into a more compassionate and loving way of relating to ourselves, for coming to a realization of deeper meaning and purpose, rests in the acceptance of where we find ourselves at this moment. At the moment when Harvey was able to say to himself that "I will cease trying to avoid and run away from what I am feeling, and I will hold up even the most impactful of feelings for listening and observation," cracks began to appear in his ego's defense armor. His life as he knew it was beginning to change. When he sets into motion the very possibility of learning from his experiences, change will happen. His bitterness towards his ex–wife will start to melt away. Why? Perhaps because he will begin to take responsibility for his part in the break up. Perhaps he will also begin to forgive himself and show compassion towards his own life. Perhaps he will see that the clock cannot be turned back and as long as he stays angry and bitter, he will be the one hurting himself, not his ex–wife. Whatever Harvey's learning will be, one thing is certain – he will become freer inside to make positive choices about how he wants his future to be. His soul will get in balance with his ego. His world will change. If we do not become willing to learn, we allow those feelings of blame, anger and bitterness to continue to gain strength and energy. Instead of bringing the life of the soul to bear on life's experiences, some people "choose" forms of addictive behavior to help them forget or cope. The consequences of not caring for ourselves can become workaholism, drug and alcohol addiction, and gambling.

If we can learn to stay connected to the power of our soul in the face of anger, bitterness, or rage, then we will be in a position to create a context of learning from the experience. Our internal activity results in meaning and purpose. They are our soul's gift to our conscious self that gives us the energy to continue doing what we are called to do. For a physician like Harvey, he is beginning to see that his work, his practice, is a vocation. It is a place where he is called to live out his spiritual journey.

Working with rather than struggling against unwanted experiences and feelings in our life is not accomplished through a problem–solving approach, the characteristic approach in training physicians in practicing the science of medicine.

Stop and think about this statement for a moment: we become like the "enemy" our mind has created and judged to be so. Perhaps that "enemy" is our spouse, a leader at the hospital, our direct supervisor, a department head, a politician, or anyone else who seems to cause anger or resentment in our life? The defense mechanism that our ego employs to justify its existence and keep us from dealing with our life experiences is called projection. Clinically, the notion of projection states that whatever we have not fully accepted within ourselves gets projected out unconsciously onto another. The only thing that can stop the dynamic of projection is conscious awareness that what we criticize in someone else is really the very thing we have not accepted in ourselves.

I stayed in contact with Harvey over a period of time. During one of our times together, I asked him this question around the bitterness he felt towards his ex–wife, "What are the things that you most criticize about her?" Harvey rattled off four things: didn't communicate well, never understood the demands of my medical practice, never appreciated all the work I do and the standard of living that my medical practice provides, and turned my children against me. I then asked this question, "What in your attitude or behavior is like that which you criticize in her?" At first Harvey denied that he was even remotely like his ex–wife. I encouraged him to walk with these two questions for a few days in an honest and open way. A week later, Harvey called and simply said, "I know now what you mean." He made the connection. His self–knowledge was enhanced once he could get his arms around where to look. The two questions became the tools for that to happen.

This process does not employ a problem solving approach wherein there are discovered solutions to an issue. Nor is this process of self–knowledge one of diagnosis, like a broken leg that can be fixed, or a virus that can be cured with antibiotics. What Harvey needed to understand is that he could not solve all the problems out there. He could not change his ex–wife, or the attitude his children had towards him, or the physician/hospital integration issues. He, as we all do, had to first acknowledge that there was something inside of himself that needed tending to. How I am with myself will determine how effectively I interact with others. Change happens when the environment, or relationship of energy between my self and others, is conducive. It is into that environment that we invite or don't invite the parties involved.

I am not naive enough to believe that there are not problems out there that need resolution. There clearly are. And some of these problems need the light of science and rational methodologies. However, what I am strongly suggesting is that we bring to the table not just our role as physician, spouse, parent, diagnostician, negotiator, et al, but also the light, energy, and power of our soul that seeks inclusion rather than exclusion in the process. For it is our soul life that seeks reconciliation rather than division, forgiveness rather than blame, freedom from the debilitating effects of anger, bitterness and rage rather than feeding and giving power to these feelings.

Self–reflection: on being here

"Stand still. The trees ahead and bushes beside you are not lost. Wherever you are is called Here, and you must treat it as a powerful stranger."

Are you able to stand still and feel your feelings and accept wherever you are at in your life's journey right now? Have there been long periods of time where you have lost your sense of purpose felt that your life was out of whack? Can you honestly say that "here" is exactly where you need to be and no where else? To what extent are you able to accept that you are called to be empowered through your experiences, not in spite of them? What is your asking of you today – and what are you asking of your life?

A walk on the wild side

Think of a time in your life when nothing seemed to go right, when debts accrued faster than income, when relationships messed up everything you tried to do, when you felt no one really understood you, when you took inventory of your life and everything was out of control. You probably felt miserable and like nothing you did made your life feel any better. You probably felt trapped. You may have felt a sense of panic, depression, anger, or resentment, and a real uncertainty about a future that seemed beyond your control. You may have wished that life would return to a simpler format. How do we live with these and similar kinds of thoughts and feelings without having them overwhelm us? When I feel like I am in that place, I remember what a wise person once shared with me: "Bill, learn to take a walk on the wild side. You are exactly where you need to be in your life." I responded, "And just where is this wild side that I need to be? And why do you say I am exactly where I need to be in my life right now? Are you nuts or what?" I said rather sarcastically. He responded, "You want the neat and predictable, a sense of control. That is your personality speaking. You are so caught up in activity, that you are forgetting who you are. That is your wild side, your soul as it interacts with each experience of your life. To listen and observe is to walk on the wild side."

A case study

Steve K. is a practicing OB/GYN in a large urban area. At 50 years of age, he has seen his practice dwindle over the past five years or so. Many of the referrals he used to get are now going to family medicine physicians. This is due in large part to insurance contracts with the large businesses that employ union labor. He still gets some of the higher risk patients. In addition, more and more women want to see female OB/GYNs. I met Steve at a conference with a group of physicians, where, in a loud and angry voice, he blamed family practice physicians for his declining practice, bemoaned the insurance companies, and became downright angry and resentful of anyone who appeared to disagree with him. During a break, one of Steve's colleagues came up to me and talked about him. This physician shared with me that Steve's marriage was on shaky ground and that his anger, blame and resentment were becoming stuff that legends are made of within the medical community. His colleagues were distancing themselves from him. Even some of the primary care physicians who were steady referral sources were sending patients elsewhere. Steve was getting more and more out of control in public forums. He was his own worst enemy. When I talked with Steve, I believe he did not have a clue that he was in trouble.

Self—reflection

Are you comfortable on the wild side? Managing our power of choice in any given moment of our life is a challenge – a sacred contract between our ego or personality (and its needs) and our soul (and its needs). The defense mechanisms of blame, rationalizing, and projection, are ways that our personality chooses (often unconsciously) to have its needs met and to have a feeling of being in control. Over time, Steve's soul life (and its needs for nourishment, reflection and prominence) retreated to a very quiet place indeed. During distressful or painful experiences, the more we try to gain control of our life, the further and further away we get from what we really want, namely, a deeper sense of meaning that is intimately connected to the life of our soul. Steve's inability to witness and observe what he was feeling through his lived experiences was causing him to react out of panic and fear rather than meaning and purpose. What experiences are causing the most distress and pain in your life? Who do you find yourself blaming when things don't go your way? How do you respond to your feelings of anger and possible resentment? How do you consciously bring the power of your soul into your everyday decisions? How comfortable are you walking on the wild side without being in control and without knowing?

How can you create more balance? True healing involves compassion and love for ourselves and others. To receive guidance from our soul and tap into its power and energy, all we need to do is to ask and then listen. Holding our life still, reflection, and inner dialogue are the playgrounds for our soul. Most of our educational systems today, especially medical education and the medical system in this country, thrive on learning new and improved ways of interacting with the outer world. The traditional medical model teaches scientific and rational ways to diagnose illness and disease. It attempts to exert positive control on the human situation. This is the world that Steve works in, where the mind–set thrives on diagnosis and control. The problem occurs when this is the only way we know and our personal life gets lived on the same wavelength as our professional training. In a realistic way, how can you bring the life of your soul and the life of your personality in alignment with each other? How would your life look if you did? How would your medical practice change if you walked on the wild side? What in you needs to change to bring more balance into your everyday living?

Your Thoughts Along The Way

*(Take a moment to write down any thoughts
or insights you want to remember.)*

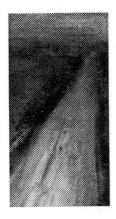

Chapter Twelve

DON'T I KNOW YOU FROM SOMEWHERE?

I am standing outside of a coffee house, gazing at the beautifully colored trees as the gentle warm breezes blow in the season of Fall. I find myself just standing there, taking in the landscape, enjoying the moment, when all of a sudden a bulldozer begins to do its thing. Beautifully colored trees, warm breezes, and a bulldozer assisting in the construction of a new mini–mall. It was a moment of contrasts.... a moment of imagination.... a moment to go back inside, sip my Colombian coffee, and let my imagination go.

A case study of sorts

Once upon a time in a land that was close to home, two perfectly matched acorns fell from the mighty oak who ruled the gentle, open farmland with loving kindness for over 80 years. The acorns had names: Joshua and Jennifer. It was time for Sean to let them go and find their own roots. Sean was a magnificent presence in the middle of the surrounding farmland, the kind of presence that gave protection from the sun's heat to the dairy cows who grazed in the pasture, and shelter to hundreds of birds who made Sean their summer home, and food to the endless numbers of squirrels who could be seen scurrying about. Sean indeed was fulfilling the calling of being an oak. Wind, rain, snow and the sun's burning heat were no match for Sean's indomitable spirit. Sean knew, you see, that the inner strength of being an oak tree depended on all the weather's elements – and I mean whatever the weather could throw at Sean – to make oak trees grow strong. Not even the Great Tornado of '46, nor the intense lightening storm of '65 could bring Sean down. The ecosystem relied on Sean's being a sturdy oak for balance to happen all around. Sean knew the secret writing within the soul of nature – let go, surrender and be stronger because of it. Sean just knew that whatever came by way of the farmland was meant for strength, energy and growth into beauty.

It now became Jennifer and Joshua's turn to germinate and create new life. They had been blown by the strong midwestern winds to spots equidistant from Sean – about 40 yards I'd say to the right and to the left. The rains came and the sun drenched the two acorns as they each began to develop the roots that would continue growing deeper into the good earth. Their destiny of continuing the legacy of being an oak tree depended as much on the cooperating ecosystem as it did on the potential of the essential oak nature inside of them. Sean soon became their mentor, protector, and friend. As the tallest tree for as far as the eye could see, Sean teased the wind, laughed at the lightening strikes nearby, and thanked Mother Earth for another day of life. Jenny and Josh (as Sean liked to call them I am told) grew in age and strength as the years passed by. They learned the wisdom of being an oak from their teacher. Each in their own way responded to the demands of the environment and the changes that being an oak tree in a rich, verdant pasture had brought. Artists and poets would give witness in paint and pen to Sean, Jenny and Josh as they fulfilled the journey required of them, a journey that began in seed. Indeed, the quiet farmland was enriched by the presence of this trinity of oaks whose commanding status was in sharp contrast to the flatness of the land.

The story line shifts to 1987 and I remember saying to myself, "I wonder if the golden age of being a stately oak tree is over!" I visit Sean, Jenny and Josh often, whenever I feel like I need to hold my own life quiet and still and allow my own roots to be nourished. But now, instead of the vast open countryside, I see subdivisions sprouting up all over the land. Our community of three oaks is now competing for space and attention by competing developers, each trying to outdo the other with the rapidity of their expansion efforts. No one seems to remember that Sean has been a nurturing presence in that field for nearly 140 years, Jenny and Josh for over 70 years. At first blush, tradition seems to be taking a back seat to progress, or at least what some call progress!

Josh speaks first, "What have you done for me lately? That's all these idiots care about. Growth, expansion, making money! Get a life, will ya? I've been around for 70 years, I was here first anyway."

Sean listens and senses the anger and bitterness in Josh as he burrows more deeply and stridently into the earth for the long road ahead. Sean compassionately responds, "It sounds, Josh, like you don't want to go down without a fight. Have you given any thought to the premise that there might be another way that will not do violence to your nature? It might be worth exploring alternatives – or is stubbornness your only ally now? You still have choices, you know, about your place in the universe."

Jenny, to Sean's right side, talks softly with Sean during the time of night when oak trees are given the gift of speech and can communicate with their peers. (I know this to be true because their roots, their oak souls, are intertwined deep beneath the earth knowing that, in the scheme of things, they share a common destiny.) Jenny's leaves for the first time in recent memory have begun to droop in the middle of the summer. The sap running throughout her veins has slowed down and only with a great degree of difficulty can get to her outer extremities. That life force impelling her towards being a stately oak seems to be sagging and retreating to a quiet place within her.

This has not gone unnoticed by Sean who quietly speaks to her, "Don't ever forget from whence you came. Oakness may take different forms after all is said and done, but all these new forms are meant to serve life, the larger, meaningful life of the ecosystem. That is our destiny, our journey together. All we can do is allow our oakness to serve life. It's part of the Plan."

Some time went by. Just as Jenny listened and become more beautiful during this turbulent time, so Josh became stiffer, more belligerent. Jenny took Sean's heartfelt advice and with Sean as her mentor developed a deep sense of surrender to the Plan. (I know this to be true, because I was there and heard it!)

"Our journeys, our destinies, have been part of us since we were wee little acorns!" said Sean. It is as if they were written into our oak souls from the moment we let go and fell from Mother Tree." Sean paused a moment, and then added, "Josh, let go. As oaks, we cannot always control what is happening all around us. No one can. We cannot control what others do or don't do. We cannot control the movements of the larger social ecosystem. What we can do is to cooperate in strength."

"When it comes right down to it, we are what we are. Our freedom is in responding, in choosing how we respond, not passively, but actively, to what Life offers as food for our souls. Therein lies our meaning and purpose for being oaks and not pine trees, or fish or rabbits. We were appointed and called to be oaks from all time, Josh. Breathe in the magnificent sunlight, bring it down deep into your roots. Relish the rain by opening your bark and root ends to its nourishment. Thank the wind for blowing off the dead leaves and live acorns so new life can rise up once again. Please remember, and don't ever forget, that your form has already changed from a tiny acorn into a stately, strong oak! Your form will change again and it will be ok, even desired. Trust in your oakness. It is meant to serve life. Being out here in the ever-dwindling farmlands is not the only form to which our destinies are calling us. Allow transformation to happen. Choose it and you allow new and deeper levels of meaning to unfold into consciousness."

Josh asked one final time in the middle of the night when the bulldozers were quiet and the developers were at home with their families, "Sean, is it too late for me to change? Jenny seems to be doing so well. I am so deeply rooted in what I have been for some 70 years that I'm beginning to question, and doubt, whether I even have the capacity to change. Jenny is not resisting the strong winds of change, but rhythmically going with them. I, on the other hand, have been resisting all along, so much so that my branches are falling off with each new wind that blows. Jenny's suppleness sure mirrors back to me my own rigidity. Can I really change, Sean?"

Sean, knowing this would be their last night together as oak trees, simply said to his two friends, "Yes, Josh, you have the capacity to change. You and Jenny both carry within you the power to be transformed. Breathe deeply from inside your roots, and pull up the power and energy of being an oak and the awareness of deeper meaning that will be open to you. Allow your destiny to unfold. Trust the process. Do you remember how naturally you did that when you both were acorns? You trusted in the Wisdom of the Universe. The Plan's will is not done to us; it is accomplished through us. Our form may well change, but our identity of who we are will not."

The winds blew hard for the next several weeks. Upon returning to the field after many months away, I was astonished, not by what I saw, but by what I did not see. No Sean, Jenny or Josh. I cried, I grieved my loss, I accepted, and I still believed what I remembered Sean saying, "Stay rooted in your oakness. It will take on many forms in a lifetime. But you still will be an oak, rich in meaning and purpose, fulfilling your destiny according to the Plan."

The time is March, 1996, and I am sitting at home in the family room. It is 2:00 in the morning and I can't sleep. Sam and Jessie are fast asleep, cuddled up with their favorite stuffed animals. I gaze out the window and focus my mind's eye on the place Sean, Jenny and Josh used to be. I give thanks for their memory. I listen and observe the moment as I hold my life still. The winds are calm now, only an occasional car interrupts the silence of this moment. I begin to hear familiar voices coming from the kitchen, a place of nourishment, family gathering, conversation and laughter. I begin to hear the table come alive and whisper to the chairs, "Don't I know you from somewhere?" I remembered that this was the time of the night that oaks could speak!

I went off to bed smiling. A deep sense of knowing and trusting filled my heart and mind. I do believe in miracles. I believe in a participating Universe where I, like Sean, Josh and Jenny, are not just observers of change. I believe that I, like all of us, participate in a Universe that calls me, and us, to be co–creators of a reality that goes to the soul of the matter.

To contact Bill Bazan, please call or write him at:

> 11925 West Lake Park Drive, Suite 100
> Milwaukee, WI   53224
> 414.359.1783
> or e mail **bbazan@mailbag.com**

For more information on the *Medicine in Search of Meaning* program, please contact:

> Bonnie Kartman, Operations Director
> Catholic Health Association of Wisconsin
> 5721 Odana Road
> Madison, WI 53719-1222
>
> 608.274.5588
> e mail **bkartman@execpc.com**